A GRACEFULLY FOR WOMEN OVER 50

DR. STEVE'S GUIDE TO HELP REVERSE AGING, DISEASE, WEIGHT GAIN, AND ENERGY LOST

DR. STEVE KRINGOLD

DEDICATION

This book is dedicated to my wife, Debra. Without your unwavering support, sacrifice, and belief in me, this work would not be possible. You taught me the true meaning of love and turned all the challenges that came our way into adventures that made our partnership thrive.

And to the ever-increasing number of women who are concerned about the effects of Aging, and how they can prevent, delay, and reverse the process through education, understanding and commitment.

JUST FOR YOU!

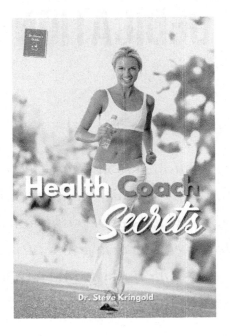

A SPECIAL GIFT FOR OUR READERS

Included with your purchase of this book is a special bonus I want you to have, which will help you on your journey to Aging Gracefully in the best of health. Please click the link below to get this important addition.

You'll receive my Health Coach Secrets book which includes:

Diet tips to help you eat clean, an emotional eaters guide, managing food cravings, with chapters on processed foods, grains, and sugar detox. You'll also be getting my macronutrients training guide and my 21 days move well program for balance and fitness.

Click the URL below to receive!

https://dashboard.mailerlite.com/forms/66438/58708344279401478/share

CONTENTS

INTRODUCTION

> *You don't stop laughing when you grow old, you grow old when you stop laughing.*
> **–George Bernard Shaw**

Growing older isn't always pleasant; the aches and pains only remind us of our mortality. But I like to think about the positive side of aging and always tell myself that they call it 'growing' older for a reason.

With age comes wisdom, as they say, and that is one hundred percent true. Years and years of self-discovery has made us more emotionally resilient. This inner strength brings with it the ability to accept that everyone ages—it's a fact of life. It is up to us to make sure we age gracefully.

That is why I decided to write this book. I had been a doctor for many years (now retired for almost 30 years) and throughout my medical career, countless women have walked into my office with the same concerns about growing older. It is as if the realization that they're not as young as they used to be had hit them overnight. It makes sense if you consider that a woman's focus is very rarely on herself; she has kids to raise, a husband to care for, and in many cases, a career to build. There's hardly any time left to think about getting older and before she knows it, she's looking at herself in the mirror and doesn't fully recognize the woman staring back.

Now that her children have left the nest and she's nearing retirement, she can start to focus on herself again. It's then that she wants to improve her overall health and well-being. Of course, this is only one example. There's no single type of woman who experiences the desire to delay aging and feel younger; it is a universal longing, as is the feeling of not knowing what to do and where to start to improve their health.

Since you're reading *Aging Gracefully for Women over 50,* I am sure you resonate with what you've read so far and are looking for someone to guide you in aging gracefully. Well, let me introduce myself: I am Dr. Steve Kringold, and I am passionate about reversing the aging process and associated diseases. I specialized in foot and ankle surgery, sports medicine, and wound care. I am a member of the American Academy of Anti-Aging Medicine, and although retired for many years, I want to help women such as yourself feel better about themselves.

There are just under 109 million people aged 50 and up in America, and more than half of this number is made up of women (AARP, 2014). You can take solace in knowing that You're not the only one going through this. Countless women worry about looking younger for longer, but most importantly, are concerned about their health as their body grows older.

We're going to take a holistic approach to making you feel as good about yourself as possible. That means we'll have a look at what you're eating, how you're sleeping, what you're doing to stay active, and what you're thinking and feeling—all important aspects that contribute to your overall health. I'll share with you some simple, yet highly effective methods you can use to make changes in your life that will lead to you looking and feeling younger.

I had a patient named Doris, many years ago, who had walked into my office totally distraught. She went to a mother-and-daughter dinner and couldn't help but notice how other women seemed to age more gracefully. This triggered a slew of emotions with anger leading the pack. She was angry at herself for "letting herself go."

I'm going to tell you what I had told Doris: It's not about letting yourself go; it's about time and gravity. There's no escaping getting older and yes, while there are ways you can look and feel better as you age, nothing you do will be able to stop the aging process entirely. The sooner you make peace with that, the easier it will be for you to focus on making the changes that will improve your quality of life as you grow.

The biggest mistake Doris made was comparing herself to others. That is opening the door to insecurity and self-doubt, which will only make you feel worse about yourself. Instead of comparing yourself, admire other women instead. If you see someone the same age as you, but they look younger, don't get jealous. This is about your journey—not theirs. Remember, their genetics may be more forgiving, or maybe they had work done; you never know, so don't assume you did something wrong and that that is why you have a wrinkle or two more or weigh a few pounds extra.

Mindset is such a vital part of aging gracefully; it's often neglected. When you look at anti-aging articles in magazines, there is a big focus on diet and exercise. Although these two aspects are just as important, when you're not in the right frame of mind, it is going to be very hard to commit to eating healthy and moving your body regularly. It goes without saying that there will be a big emphasis on fostering and maintaining a positive mindset in this book. In fact, since I believe mindset is the foundation for everything this book is based on, it is appropriate to kick off with it.

Before we move on to Chapter 1, I want to remind you that although I am a doctor, I don't know your medical history. I'm not aware of any medical conditions you may have or are predisposed to. For this reason, consult with your doctor before making any major changes that can negatively affect your health. I have also been retired for the past 25 years, but still attend medical conferences as an active member of the American

Academy of Anti-Aging Medicine and continue to read the latest in medical journals and articles. My aim is to improve your health, not make it worse, so please approach this book with your body and well-being in mind.

CHAPTER 1:
A MINDSET OF CHANGE

There's something we need to establish before we continue: You're not "over the hill" when you turn 50. There are wonderful benefits to reaching this milestone.

Yes, you may have dark circles under your eyes and gray hairs popping up faster than you can get an appointment at your hairstylist but remember one thing: Growing older is a privilege that not everyone gets to experience.

No one is asking you to deny the more undesirable aspects of getting older, but maybe thinking about the positives as well will balance out your feelings about aging.

So, let's start changing your viewpoint about life over 50.

Your Self-Confidence Improves

When You're younger, you tend to be conscious about your flaws and worry more about what other people think of you. A lot of women have noted growing grateful for their flaws as they aged. To them, every scar and every wrinkle tells the story of their life and holds memories they don't want to forget. This realization caused them to stop comparing themselves to others. It is genuinely a freeing experience.

It's Easier for You to Say No

Saying yes to things you don't want to do can bring you down and drain your energy. Luckily, once you turn 50, you'll find it much easier to say no. Your time becomes precious, and you don't want to waste it on anything That's not worth it. The ease of setting boundaries and sticking to them as you grow older is a wonderful thing—it's a great way to protect your health, both physical and mental.

Your Priorities Change

When you turn 50, the things you felt were important in your 20's no longer are. Some women realize there are more valuable things to do with their time than ticking swimming with sharks or bungee jumping off their bucket list. On the flip side, other women may consider these very things as important and set out to do them, instead of doing things that are considered more age appropriate.

You're Wiser

You gained a lot of experience in 50 years. Mistakes were made, but lessons were also learned along the way. You can share this knowledge with your children or with anyone else who may need some guidance. That's a brilliant way to pay it forward as the wisdom you share with others may prevent them from making the same mistakes you made and avoid them having the same regrets.

You Criticize Yourself Less

One of my past patients described reaching 50 as a light bulb moment. She said she grasped that she was good enough all of a sudden. Yes, she still wanted to lose those extra pounds, but she wasn't going to wait around and put life on hold until she lost the weight. Your happiness shouldn't depend on how you look, what you own, or anything else That's trivial. Thankfully, that is something you realize as you grow older. It's easier to be at peace with things that once bothered you.

You're Willing to Take Risks

If there was ever a time to take risks, it's now. When we're young, we have many 'tomorrows' and 'laters', but when you turn 50, it dawns on you that there's no need (or time) to wait for a special occasion to do the things you enjoy. You made it this far and are more than welcome to reward yourself by doing what you want when you want. You can be pretty sure that you won't gamble on things that can backfire and affect the remainder of your life negatively.

It's Not All About the Money Anymore

You wake up one day and acknowledge that you reached the halfway mark to the finishing line. I know it sounds somewhat morbid, but some of my past female patients had described it as a freeing feeling. They mentioned how the realization that the hourglass is running out changed their mindset from making money to spending more time with loved ones. It's not about material things anymore, but about making family and friends a top priority.

Those are only some of the benefits of turning 50 and I hope after reading this you feel a little more positive about reaching this milestone in your life. If You're not quite there yet, don't worry; at the end of this chapter, I have a suspicion that you'll embrace your age with open arms.

Positive Aging

If I were to ask you how you feel about growing old, you would undoubtedly tell me you're scared when confronted with the changes your body is going through, not to mention the realization that we're all mortal beings. Maybe You're feeling lonely as you face the reality of growing older. Whatever the case may be, it doesn't need to be that way. Positive aging helps one navigate these expected and unexpected changes gracefully

But what exactly is positive aging?

It's an interesting question, and one with varying answers. Cultures around the world don't define it the same way. For example, one culture may revere their elders, while the other values youth and physical beauty over the wisdom that comes with age.

If you grow up in a culture where a lot of emphasis is placed on outer beauty, you may fight against aging and do whatever it takes to stay young. They may even believe that aging is a disease that is curable.

In my view, it is a much better approach to accept that aging is inevitable. Your mental health (and wallet) will thank you for it.

The Psychology of Growing Older

Aging isn't always comfortable to accept. Your body is not working as it used to; aches and pains are the norm, your eyesight has weakened, and you now have to be extra careful not to fall or you might end up with a broken bone. All this undoubtedly has a psychological impact on us, especially if you grew up in a culture that worships the young and beautiful and discards the elderly.

It's not always easy to know where we belong as we grow older. The places where we used to fit in, we end up feeling out of sorts when we reach 50. We're forced to redefine who we are, and at times, find a new life's purpose. Then there's the fear of disease or worsening disease that is part and parcel of aging. When disease is so severe that outside help is needed to manage day-to-day activities, it's possible to feel frustrated and angry.

Considering the above, it's no surprise an estimated 15 million middle-aged, and older, adults will need mental and behavioral care (American Psychological Association, n.d.). There are a lot of factors contributing to anxiety and depression.

A study done by geropsychologists looked at the concept of successful aging from a cultural perspective (Martin et al., 2015). They focused on the various theories throughout history that contributed to the psychological concept of positive aging. Let me share with you some noteworthy truth-seekers who contributed to the forming of what we, today, consider positive aging.

> **Carl Jung** believed late life is the perfect time to self-reflect and look inward (Gottberg, 2015).

> **Bernice Neugarten** agreed with Jung, but later broadened her definition to include a focus on personality type in successful aging (Neugarten, 1996).

> **Erik Erikson** formulated eight stages of development, the last one being integrity versus despair. Martin sums up the eight stages as assessing one's life and coming to the conclusion that it has been fulfilling and satisfying. This would then be considered successful aging.

> **Robert Havighurst** coined the term "successful aging" (Havighurst, 1961). He focused on satisfaction and happiness. According to him, aging is active or

disengaging. Active aging is when a person carries over middle-aged activities and attitudes to an older age. Disengaged aging, on the other hand, is when someone tries to remove themselves from leading an active and engaging life.

These are only some definitions of positive or successful aging throughout the decades. You can see that there's a golden thread woven throughout all these classifications: one of peace and fulfillment. I think that is one of my main goals in writing this book. I want you to take on the coming years with a feeling of serenity, working with your body as it ages and not against it.

To help you achieve such a level of acceptance, we first need to look at the negative beliefs about aging, and why you shouldn't pay much mind to them.

Negative Beliefs About Aging

There are various unchallenged beliefs about aging entrenched in society. These stereotypes can affect a person's self-perception. When it comes to aging, there are quite a few negative stereotypes that you need to leave behind if you want to age gracefully. For example, when you think of older people, how do you picture them? I won't be surprised if the words: frail, slow, and forgetful come to mind. Sickly, inept, helpless, and weak probably also popped into your head. These are adjectives many people use to describe anyone over 50.

These contribute heavily to the negativity women experience around aging, which is unfortunate as the wealth of knowledge that comes with growing older gets overshadowed. What's more, the pervasiveness of these stereotypes in Western culture can affect how older adults recover from disease (Dionigi, 2015).

In 2016, the World Health Organization (WHO) conducted a global survey to measure the amount of discrimination older adults experience. The survey found that 60% of older respondents don't feel respected. Interestingly, the elderly from high-income countries experienced the lowest level of respect. Furthermore, the survey echoed Dionigi's findings above: The negativity surrounding aging contributes to ill health.

In a study titled "You're Only as Old as You Feel" (2016), researchers found that seniors with a negative attitude toward aging walked slower than their positive counterparts. But what's worse, they also had worse cognitive abilities down the line. The conclusion is that negative perceptions of growing older can affect frontal cognitive domains in the elderly (Robertson & Kenny, 2016).

If you're still not convinced that your attitude impacts how well you age, let me offer you Alice Herz-Sommer as an example. She survived the Holocaust and won her battle against cancer to live to the age of 110 years old. How? Well, according to her, "Everything in life is a present." Now if that isn't a positive attitude, I don't know what is!

If you're wondering how you can foster a more positive attitude towards aging, National Geographic fellow Dan Buettner may have part of the answer for you. He discovered five places in the world where people live the longest and healthiest lives. He dubbed this the Blue Zone and it includes, Okinawa, Japan; Sardinia, Italy; Nicoya, Costa Rica; Ikaria, Greece; and Loma Linda, California (Blue Zones, n.d.). Also, with the help of demographers and researchers, he discovered nine lifestyle habits practiced by people living in the Blue Zones.

1. Move More

People who live in the Blue Zones are naturally more active. They are forced to move without thinking about it too much. Exercise for them isn't so much going to the gym, but natural workouts like walking or gardening.

2. Have Purpose

The Japanese call it 'ikigai,' meaning life's purpose. You need a reason to get up in the morning. If you find it, you may increase your lifespan by as much as seven years (Positive Psychology, 2022).

3. Take It Down a Notch

People in the Blue Zones know how to manage their stress. They meditate, take a lot of naps, and generally try to lead a stress-free life.

4. Control Your Weight

The secret to a longer life may be as simple as to stop eating before you're full. It also works if you eat your largest meal early in the day and keep it light in the early evening.

5. Magic Beans

People in the Blue Zones don't eat a lot of meat. They mainly eat fish as their protein source, some chicken, and pork a few times a month. They do, however, eat a lot of fruit and vegetables; beans are a solid favorite.

6. Have a Drink

There's no need to feel shame if you enjoy a glass of red every night. In fact, Buettner found that everyone (except Adventists) in the Blue Zone enjoyed alcohol. They drank 1–2 glasses a day.

7. Belong

Be part of a faith-based community. Beuttner's research found that attending religious services four times per month could add between 4–14 years to your life.

8. Put Your Family First

There is a big focus on family in the Blue Zones. You'll find that parents and grandparents live together with their children, or in close proximity. This decreases mortality rates and lowers the risk of disease.

9. Choose Who You Surround Yourself With

If you have a supportive social circle, they'll root for you when you make good life decisions. So, make sure to spend your time with the right people.

As you can see, positive aging is all about adopting a positive stance on growing older. It's about seeing it as a healthy and normal part of life and using the time you have left to do the things you love.

There are many things you gain as you grow older. I recommend you make a list of the good things about reaching 50. Then, when you feel despondent about your age, refer to your list to get a little perspective.

If I had to write a list, I would include:

> ➤ I have more time to spend with my grandchildren.

> ➤ I can go on walks more often.

> ➤ I can spend time on my favorite hobbies.

> ➤ I'm able to learn a new skill.

These are only some of the encouraging things about getting older. I'm sure you can relate to some of them and can add many more reasons to appreciate your golden years. If you're not quite there yet, there are ways to get rid of that negative voice that keeps pointing out all the unpleasant aspects of aging.

First, we have to fully understand what negative self-talk is before we do something about it.

Negative Self-Talk: First Step to Failure

The less-than-desirable thoughts running through your mind aren't helping you. You may wake up some days thinking You're entitled to bemoan your lot, and on some days, it may be just what you need. You know, get it out of your system and move on. It becomes a problem when you wallow in negative self-talk.

What you must remember is that this type of internal dialogue doesn't just stay in your mind; it can lead to actions that you may regret. You may refuse an opportunity because you don't think you're worthy—you're too old and over the hill—only to later realize that it was something you truly wanted. I can give you myriad examples of how negative thoughts permeate every aspect of your life.

Unfortunately, negative self-talk can be a very comfortable place. Yes, you may put yourself down, but at least you're not putting yourself out there. You're not opening yourself up for possible ridicule, judgment, and heartache if you lock yourself in your house with your negative thoughts, right? Although that may be true, that is not living; that is hiding. If you give in to your negative feelings, you're allowing it to steal—it's stealing your attention, your happiness, and your time.

There's no time for you to focus on the present when you're stuck in the past. You also can't be happy when everything that fills your mind is negative. In time, this negativity consumes you until you have no hopes and you're blind to all opportunities for better things.

Do you understand how this frame of mind is the first step to failure? It gets you in its grip and will keep you trapped there unless you do something to break free. If you don't, fear of what could happen as you age, stress over what you need to do to prepare for death, and frustration over the unfairness of aging will bring you down and you'll spend your last years gripped in sadness.

I remind you of Alice Herz-Sommer, a woman who faced unspeakable odds but always looked for the silver lining. There are many other examples of people who had to overcome unrealistic odds, but they ended up making the best of it and succeeded. On the other hand, you get those who were given every opportunity in life but ended up miserable. This goes to show that whatever your circumstances are, your attitude determines your response and that influences the outcome.

I also want you to realize that you're not born positive. Humans are hardwired with negative emotions. It is how we survived as hunter-gatherers and humans predating the Neolithic agricultural revolution (McMahon, 2017). Humans had no choice but to constantly scan the world for threats. Although many of us don't have to worry about food scarcity, shelter, and all other basic human needs anymore, our brains adapt, and they will still choose to entertain negative thoughts over positive ones. The good news is, you *can* reprogram your brain to be more optimistic, and ultimately, change it so that your inner voice is more compassionate when you look in the mirror.

Getting there, however, is not a straight path. There's no off switch for negative self-talk, so there will be times when harmful thoughts slip through. That is why it is extremely important that we're mindful of the words we use. The better you get at noticing negative self-talk, the easier it will become to deal with these types of thoughts and change them into positive ones.

The difficulty lies in recognizing negative self-talk. Here's a breakdown of the four main types in order for you to know what to look out for.

Personalizing

There's this "It's not you; it's me" joke people make when it comes to breakups. In the case that it is the other person, but you still choose to use this line, you're personalizing. Basically, you blame yourself for something bad even though you're not in the wrong.

Another example would be when your friend doesn't text you for a while and you think they're mad at you or don't want to be friends anymore. The fact that they might just be busy doesn't even cross your mind.

To beat this type of negative thinking, you must do a reality check.

Stop and ask yourself:

> ➤ What evidence is there to support what I'm thinking?
> ➤ Are my thoughts based on facts or is it my personal interpretation?

Now think of an alternative reason that offsets your negative thoughts.

In the event that you're blaming yourself for something, take a step back. It helps to look at the situation from the outside. You've been friends with this person for 25-odd years. If you didn't have a fight, there's no reason they'd suddenly stop liking you. Are there any more logical reasons why they haven't answered your texts? Yes! You forgot they have an important meeting to prepare for and have been doing mountains of research might be one of them.

Filtering

Think of filtering as a magnifying glass that enlarges only the negative parts of a situation. A good example is when you put on your favorite pair of jeans, but the button won't close; this is something that happens with a lot of women as they get older. A common reaction is to spiral down into despair as the words: fat, ugly, and undesirable come to mind. You forget that your friend complimented you on your hair a few days ago and that your partner told you how beautiful you looked yesterday. What about the two pounds you lost last week because you've been watching your diet and exercising more?

Whenever you catch yourself filtering, grab a piece of paper and write down all the good things surrounding the situation. As the list keeps growing, you'll slowly recognize that things truly aren't as bad as you feel they are. You may even remember that you ate onion last night and now you're a little bloated!

Catastrophizing

You're on your way to the office and find yourself in the middle of some bad traffic. The first thing you think is, "I'm going to be stuck here for hours." You're catastrophizing by instinctively anticipating the worst.

When this happens, try to get some perspective. Consider other outcomes and try to distinguish between what is really possible and what isn't. Is it possible for traffic on the freeway to come to a complete halt for hours? If so, what is the worst that would happen and what steps can you take to lessen the impact? If you're worried you'll be late for work, phone your boss and let them know. They'll probably be aware of the traffic jam and may even be stuck in it themselves.

Polarizing

If you experience life as black and white with no gray area, then you're polarizing. You're either perfect or you're a failure; there's no middle ground.

Let's say you decide to go on a diet because you want to lose a few pounds. You've been sticking to your eating plan for two weeks, but one day you struggle and end up eating a slice of cake. Instead of acknowledging your success of the previous weeks, you focus on today and feel like a failure. This type of negative self-talk has the power to demotivate you because you end up being too hard on yourself.

If you catch yourself polarizing situations, treat yourself with kindness. Remind yourself that you're human and you're not perfect. You will make mistakes, but you will learn from them and do better next time.

You'll have to put on your boxing gloves to fight negative self-talk. It takes a lot of practice as negativity is extremely hard to shake. I always use to tell my patients to practice positivity every second of the day. Don't wait until you recognize a negative thought to ramp up the optimism. Get a head start by repeating some positive affirmations as soon as you wake up. Tell yourself that you've got this and challenge yourself to find the good in any negative thought that may pop into your head throughout the day.

It's all about acknowledging that for every problem, there usually is a solution. I don't want you to disregard the bad in any situation; I want you to trust that you'll find a way around it.

Consequences of Negative Self-Talk

Our internal dialogue doesn't only affect how we feel about ourselves, but it can impact our mental health and can trigger depression and other mental health diseases (Kinderman et al., 2013).

When you entertain negative self-talk for a prolonged period, you become stressed. It makes sense since You're constantly creating a reality where very little is possible. This can be extremely demotivating, which can lead to a feeling of helplessness as you struggle to notice opportunities, and if you do happen to see them, your negative thoughts keep you from acting on them. It's a draining cycle that will continue until you give up all hope and believe your harmful inner dialogue.

Other consequences include:

> **You limit your abilities.** You can only tell yourself you can't do something so many times before you start believing it.

> **You continue to strive for perfection.** Somewhere along the line, you must realize not many things in life are perfect. If you don't, you'll continue to believe that perfection is attainable when in reality it isn't.

➤ **You'll harm your relationships.** When you fall victim to negative self-talk regularly, you probably come across as needy and insecure. The constant self-criticism that goes hand in hand with harmful internal dialogue leads to behavior that bothers others. They may avoid talking to you as you automatically put a negative spin on everything. This is detrimental to relationships as we all know it is built on communication.

Thankfully, there are strategies you can use to quiet that over-critical voice inside your head.

Let's look at the various approaches you can take and find the best line of attack for you.

Spot the Critic and Give It a Name

Learn to recognize when you're being too hard on yourself. When you catch yourself being overly critical, stop and ask yourself if you'd talk to a friend or family member in such a manner. If your answer is no, then you shouldn't be talking to yourself this way either.

It also helps to give your inner critic a name. Ever heard of Debbie Downer? What about Negative Nelly? When you name your inner critic, you give it its own identity. This makes it more comfortable to say, "Hey, listen here, Brenda Bummer, I'm not going to listen to you." I know it may sound silly, but that's exactly what we want. The aim is to turn something threatening into a goofy character just as ridiculous as the critical thoughts we have.

Stick to Reality

Your thoughts and feelings aren't always true. You may experience them as good judgment, but they shouldn't be considered accurate without digging a little deeper. Thoughts and feelings can be skewed; they're often subject to prejudices and are influenced by our moods. So don't take them at face value.

Set Boundaries

You can give your negativity limits. When you find yourself thinking disapproving thoughts, contain the damage and tell yourself that you're only to criticize specific aspects of your life. Creating this boundary controls the amount of negativity you'll experience daily. To take it a step further, you can limit being negative to only an hour a day.

Change Your Language

It's not always easy to stop negative thoughts in their tracks. Instead of letting it steam-roll over you, try to change the power of your language. When you find yourself thinking, "I can't do this," modify it to, "This is hard." Instead of saying, "I hate," say, "I dislike," and turn down the level of negativity immediately.

Question Your Thoughts

What makes negative self-talk so prevailing is that it is often left unchallenged. It's not like those close to you are privy to your thoughts and can tell you that your thinking is wrong; You're the only one who can determine how true your thoughts are, so cross-examine your inner critic. You'll find that most of the time, your negative self-talk amplifies a situation. Stopping yourself from doing this will minimize the damaging impact of such harmful inner discourse. An example is when you think, "I haven't amounted to anything." Question if that is correct. Think about where you started in your career and where you are now. If you don't have a career, think about your children and what a dedicated mother you are.

Be Your Own Friend

We're our own worst enemies at times. How many instances have you said things to yourself in your head that you'd never say to anyone else? You must learn to treat yourself with the same kindness and compassion. One way to do this is to ask yourself if this is something you'd say to someone you cherish. Go as far as imagining yourself saying it to someone you love. I imagine you feel guilty for even thinking about treating them in such a manner. Remember this when you're not being nice to yourself. Being your own friend is a great way to keep your self-talk in check.

Change Your Perspective

Will what is upsetting you now matter tomorrow, in a month, or in the next five years? Answering this question will shift your perspective—you may realize that you're worried about much of nothing.

Another way I like to get perspective is by reminding myself that I'm only a tiny speck in a huge universe. Any negative dialogue can't compete with the vastness of such a thought, and the fear and urgency I feel for whatever reason disappears.

Talk to Yourself

Voice your negative thoughts out loud. You'll be surprised how ridiculous your negative self-talk is when said out loud. Even whispering them can make you realize how unreasonable you're being. So don't be afraid of talking to yourself. I do it often, much to the amusement of my wife and children.

Snap Out of It

Psychologists call it 'thought-stopping' and it is a technique used to prevent negative thoughts from ballooning into a full-blown anxiety or panic attack. You can use a rubber band to 'snap' yourself out of it, or you can visualize a stop sign when negative thoughts enter your mind. There are many methods you can choose from, but the general idea is to stop negative thoughts in their tracks. Thought stopping is especially helpful for those extremely critical thoughts that keep coming over and over again.

Negative self-talk doesn't have to control your life. You don't have to approach aging in any other way than with optimism and confidence. I realize it is easier said than done when faced with the harsh reality of growing older, but if you consider that a positive attitude leads to better health and mental well-being, then you have the power to increase your quality of life and life expectancy significantly.

I can't stress the influence of daily affirmations enough. Speaking a few kind words to yourself has the potential to change what you think and feel about life over 50. It makes you appreciate the good that comes with growing older. Before you know it, you won't focus on the toll that gravity is taking on your body, or the fact that you're more vulnerable to disease. Instead, your attention will be on the amount of strength your body still has, your health, and all the days filled with love and laughter you have to look forward to. What's more, the gratitude you'll feel as you concentrate on the good in your life will quiet negative self-talk further (Altman, 2019). Soon, you'll change your life's charge from negative to positive as you break the cycle of criticism and replace it with gratitude.

Meditation: The Anti-Aging Miracle

One day, while walking through our local shopping mall, my wife wandered into a cosmetics store. I followed her and was surprised with the amount of products on the shelf. Anti-wrinkle face cream, collagen-boosting night cream, anti-aging day cream, and many other concoctions. Now, as a man, I don't know much about cosmetics, and I quickly found myself utterly confused by the number of available options on the shelves. Anti-age this; anti-wrinkle that. One thing is sure, women are looking for ways to stop the aging process to achieve everlasting beauty.

My wife is a retired opera singer. She loved the stage, the make-up, and the costumes. Taking care of her body and voice was part of the job and she practiced a positive, heart centered mindset regularly. The effort she put in back then is still paying off today. Of course, the fact that she continues to do this is contributing to her youthfulness and vitality.

I may not know much about skincare, but I know that mindfulness practice—in whichever form—is an anti-aging miracle. How it works is straightforward. Stress causes the cells in our bodies to age, so if we do something to combat the stress, we automatically slow down the aging process (Epel et al. 2009).

To understand what happens to our bodies when we're under stress, we must look at how our bodies evolved over the years. I previously mentioned that we were made to have negative thoughts as it is a survival mechanism. Well, stress was the driving force behind many of these negative thoughts. Our ancestors had to deal with the stress of hunting and killing huge animals, attacking enemy tribes, or fighting diseases that had no treatment or cure. This triggered the development of the fight or flight response. But what actually happens when our body enters this mode?

In general, the brain prepares for a stressful task ahead. Our brains identify potential danger and jolt the body into action; either flee or stand and fight. This causes our heart rate to speed up, our breathing gets faster, and various other processes in our bodies get activated—most of them not very favorable toward staying young (McCarty, 2016).

We don't face the same threats as our ancestors did; there's no running away from predators and no rival tribes we must battle for land. Yet, our bodies still have the same powerful response when we're in stressful situations. This is a problem because although the stress we face today is less intense, it is more frequent, which means the fight or flight response gets triggered more often. In other words, our bodies are aging faster than our ancestors did even though they lived in more treacherous times.

It's a bad joke, really. The fight or flight response is of little use to us. It's not as if you can run away or get into a fight when you have a deadline to meet. So, we're getting all of the negative of this instinctual response, but none of its benefits.

Allow me to get technical for a moment. Each chromosome in our body has a protein cap called a telomere. When the cells divide, the chromosome replicates, which shortens the telomere. There comes a point when the telomeres are too short, which prevents the cell from further division. This increases aging and causes age-related diseases.

In other words, if scientists can find a way to slow down or prevent telomeres from becoming too short, they'll effectively slow down the aging process. But, since we're not there yet, you have to do what you can to help the telomeres stay long enough to allow cell division. Leading a healthy lifestyle goes a long way to achieving this goal, but reducing stress goes even farther.

The most well-known study done on telomeres explored the effects of stress on mothers with chronically ill children (Epel et al. 2004). The results were significant. The mothers who lived in such highly stressful circumstances had shorter telomeres than the control group. Shockingly, when you put a time stamp on the shortened telomeres, the stressed mothers were approximately 10 years older than the women who didn't experience similar stressors.

That's definite proof—and only one study out of many—that stress ages our bodies.

This brings me back to meditation or mindfulness in any form. It is a known and proven stress buster! One study found that meditation can increase the length of telomeres (Conklin et al. 2018). The participants meditated for just 15 minutes daily and this increased telomerase production. What's more, the study found that any exercise that triggered relaxation, including yoga and reciting mantras, helped repair telomeres.

The benefits of meditation aren't limited to keeping you young from the inside out though. Some other advantages include:

➤ It's free. That's good news considering that anti-aging treatments tend to be very expensive.

➤ It doesn't take long. You don't have to spend hours practicing mindfulness to reap the benefits; 15 minutes a day is all you need.

➤ Your concentration will improve. Add to that increased memory and improved attention span, and your risk of getting neurological disorders as you age decreases significantly.

➤ It makes you happier, and the happier you are, the less stress you'll experience and the younger you'll feel (and look).

➤ You'll feel less anxious, and your overall emotional health will get a boost.

➤ You'll be more self-aware and will get to know yourself on a deeper level.

➤ You'll sleep better.

➤ It reduces blood pressure (Ponte Marquez et al. 2019).

➤ You can do it anywhere and at any time.

There's no way to stop stress—it is part of life as we know it. But by dealing with it in a healthier manner, you can train your brain and body to react to it less severely. The best way to do this is through mindfulness practice. It doesn't matter if you choose meditation, yoga, or a long stroll through the park, as long as it is an activity that relaxes you and brings your mind to the here and now. It is also something you have to practice daily if you want to gain all the benefits.

To help you turn your mindfulness into a habit, follow the tips below.

Pick a Time

If possible, set a specific time aside daily for your mindfulness practice. This will help you get into a routine and before you know it, it will be a habit you can't live without. Some people like to meditate or do yoga early in the morning, while others prefer to go for a relaxing walk in the afternoon. Both times of day have their pros. Meditating in the morning can help improve your focus while doing it at night will help you sleep. It truly is up to you to find out what works best in your life.

Create a Calm Space

Try to find a space that is free from distractions; no televisions, radios, phones, or the like. Make the space as comfortable as possible and try your best to do it in the same space each time. This way, as soon as you enter the room, your body and mind will start to relax in preparation for your mindfulness practice.

Make it Easy

The easier your practice is, the easier it will be to make it a habit. I find it helps to start slow. If you can only do it for two minutes, that is two minutes more than zero. So go for it! Work your way up to where you want to be. When you do it every day, you'll soon find that you can easily go for 10 or 15 minutes.

The human mind is astonishing. Many, many hours of research have gone into understanding how it works, and yet we still know so little. What we do know is that your mind has the power to harm or heal you and it's very much up to you to decide what it should do. Negative thinking can be your downfall as you enter this time of your life. It can drag you down mentally, emotionally, and physically and suck the joy out of what can be a time of adventure and self-discovery.

When you can control your mind, you'll be able to control how you experience aging. I suggest you start by getting rid of all the stereotypes of life over 50. Let go of words like frail, sickly, clumsy, useless, and any other term used to describe older people.

They say you're only as old as you feel. This is true if you consider that leading a happy and relaxed life actually affects the makeup of your cells! Now is the perfect time to challenge your beliefs about aging and create your own reality; one free from fear, worry, and disappointment. To help you get there, find a quiet spot, sit down, and close your eyes for a few minutes. The power of just being is compelling, and as you sit there, be kind to yourself. Tell yourself that you're not defined by your age or outer beauty but by the road you've traveled to get to where you are.

In the next chapter, we're going to have a look at the role diet plays in aging and what you can do to live a longer and healthier life. Don't worry, I'm not going to tell you to cut all sugar and live only on grapefruit and toast!

Chapter Summary

> Stereotypes about aging can affect your self-perception positively or negatively.

> The negativity around aging contributes to poor health.

> Your attitude impacts how you age.

> Look for the positive attributes of life over 50.

> Humans are hardwired with negative emotions, but we can reprogram our brains.

> Stress causes us to age faster.

> Mindfulness combats stress and changes the structure of your cells to keep you younger for longer.

CHAPTER 2:
FUELING YOUR BODY

How you fuel your body impacts not only how you look but how you feel. Unfortunately, many women fall for fad diets or miracle weight-loss potions and pills that leave them feeling like failures. It worked for Kim Kardashian and her sisters, so why didn't it work for you? Well, because it *didn't* work for them!

You can't compare yourself to the rich and famous who have access to daily personal trainers, meal planners, and plastic surgeons to shape their bodies. You also shouldn't trust everything you see on the internet. Shapewear and photo editing are powerful tools that make celebrities look slimmer than they truly are. I'm sure you've seen the candid and unfiltered beach shots captured by sneaky paparazzi that reveal a whole different silhouette than what the glammed-up, red carpet photos show.

The bottom line is that there's no quick fix to re-shape your body. It takes hard work and dedication. Regrettably, it's much easier and more enjoyable to put on weight than to lose it. Fad diets promise these amazing results, but the fact that they're not sustainable makes it hard to achieve the weight loss you're hoping for. If you do happen to push through, the chance that you'll gain it all back with interest is very likely. That's because fad diets don't teach you how to fuel your body; they don't explain the concept of calories in versus calories out. So, when you're done with the program, you go back to eating exactly the way you were, and in the matter of days, the number on the scale is up again and you start looking for the latest weight-loss craze to try out.

I can't tell you how many women have a history of yo-yo dieting. I have seen multiple female patients over the years who mention they're on a diet and when I see them again in a few months, they haven't lost any weight and they're on yet another diet. Popular magazines, blogs, and society in general, don't do much to rectify this issue but exacerbate it by publishing the latest fad diets. There's a massive focus on losing weight but not much medically sound information on how to do it.

In this chapter, I'll share with you all you need to know to heal your body from the inside out. When you eat wholesome foods that meet your body's energy needs, you'll feel better and look better. What and when you eat can also push the pause button on aging.

It's my hope that after you read this chapter, instead of getting excited at the latest dieting trend, you'll scoff at it because you know it won't work and the reasons why. So, let's arm you with all the knowledge you need to make the right food choices.

The Truth About Diets

"Doc, should I be on a diet?"

I've heard this question countless times. If you find yourself wondering if going on a diet is a good idea for you, here's what I say to all my patients: No.

I know this goes against what society says, and even other medical professionals, but hear me out. I hate the word 'diet' for all the reasons mentioned at the beginning of this chapter. It has been colonized by celebrities, health and fitness 'gurus,' and well-being journalists who actually know little to nothing about nutrition. Going on a diet is a short-term solution to a long-term challenge. So, you have to figure out what going on a diet means to you. Is your mission to eat as little as possible for a few days to lose X amount of weight, or do you plan on changing your relationship with food?

If the latter, then you should definitely go on a diet!

However, if you're used to restricting what you eat for a while, losing weight, gaining it back, and then finding yourself back on a diet-restarting the cycle-then you should rethink your approach.

There are many medical reasons why dieting is bad for you. For one, if you limit what you eat too much, you're restricting your body's nutrients, which means you won't get the vitamins and minerals you need.

A lack of nutrients can lead to:

> Weakness. This is especially true if you cut out carbohydrates and fat entirely (Bilsborough & Crowe, 2003). You need these essential nutrients to function.

> Hair loss. Nutritional deficiency can impact hair structure and hair growth (Guo & Katta, 2017). Without enough vitamins and minerals, the hair follicles weaken, which leads to hair fall.

But the harmful impact of dieting goes far beyond a lack of nutrients. I want to focus on two possible consequences that concern me the most.

1. Eating Disorders

Now, I realize some readers may laugh at the thought of developing an eating disorder at this time in their lives. After all, it's a teenage problem, right? No. That's not the case, and women over 50 can still experience symptoms of an eating disorder and many may relapse into habits of their younger years. In fact, the changes women go through during menopause often echo puberty, increasing the risk of developing an eating disorder. Add to those other stressors like children leaving the home (or moving back in), aging parents, and health issues, and you may not be as resilient as you'd like.

One study found that 13% of American women over 50 experience symptoms of an eating disorder and 60% are concerned about the negative effect their weight may have on their lives (Gagne et al. 2012). Even more troubling is that 70% of the participants were actively trying to lose weight.

Many women use their diet to control or deal with the negative or overwhelming feelings that go hand in hand with getting older. Regrettably, as we age, our bodies become less hardy and we're at risk of serious health complications. For women, these are exacerbated when they suffer from a midlife eating disorder. This includes a greater risk of:

➤ hormonal imbalances
➤ heart disease
➤ liver disease
➤ kidney failure
➤ osteoporosis
➤ gastrointestinal problems
➤ damage to teeth

The good news is that the maturity that comes with age can help you battle an eating disorder if you should develop one. You have more life experience and insight to understand the physical and psychological damage this behavior would have and that should help you stop before it is too late. Even women who have suffered from eating disorders earlier in their lives may find it easier to succeed this time around.

2. Muscle Loss

Lean muscles contribute to around 50% of total body weight in young adults, but as a person ages, it steadily decreases (Kalyani, Corriere, Ferrucci, 2014). When you reach 75 years, your muscle mass may be as little as 25% of your body mass. That's quite a significant drop, and one that your health practitioner will tell you to start working against as soon as you can. If you don't attempt to retain as much muscle as you can, you limit your functionality and mobility when you're older. You can't lift yourself out of bed if you don't have the muscles to do it!

Now, the reduced calorie intake that forms part of most diets can lead to a decline in muscle mass. Think of it this way, your dog is used to enjoying a full bowl of dog food every day, but you decide to cut his rations—you don't give him half of what he usually got; you give him a quarter! This goes on for a day or two. One day, you're preparing meat on the counter and turn to rinse off the veggies. When you look back, the meat is gone, and Rocky is looking at you licking his lips.

Your body is Rocky, and your muscles are the meat. When your body doesn't get its fuel from the right sources, it has no choice but to look for it elsewhere.

Throughout this section, there's a lot of focus on what you shouldn't do, but I don't want you to feel discouraged. There are things you can do to control your weight in a healthy manner. I'm a big fan of time-restricted eating. Not only does it help you lose weight while maintaining muscle, but it doesn't have to be very restrictive for you to see and feel the results. But wait, I am getting ahead of myself. I am excited to share this lifestyle with you because I know what a powerful weight-loss and anti-aging tool it is. So, let's jump right in!

Intermittent Fasting

If you've been scouring the internet for ways to lose weight, there is a very high chance that you've read about intermittent fasting (IF) before. This eating strategy has grown in popularity over the last years for its reported weight loss benefits, anti-aging effect, and physical and mental health advantages (De Cabo & Mattson, 2019).

Think of IF as an umbrella term for various fasting protocols, which we'll deal with a little later, but no matter how long you decide to fast at what time, the positive impact is undeniable.

Much of a woman's life is marred by hormones. There's the monthly cycle of estrogen and progesterone in preparation for pregnancy. These fluctuations can lead to irritability, mood swings, bloating, excessive urination, breakouts, and many other symptoms often labeled as premenstrual stress or PMS (OASH, n.d.). Then, when you do get pregnant, those hormones go into overdrive and what you experienced monthly doubles in intensity. As a bonus, you get some extra symptoms to deal with (What to expect, 2018).

Don't worry, I haven't forgotten about menopause, a time when women stop having their periods. Many readers may be heading toward menopause or may even have passed it. Menopause, with all its phases, can last up to 10 years. But no matter how long it lasts, with it comes further unwanted symptoms such as hot flashes, insomnia, sweating, and vaginal dryness (Scaccia, 2019).

Intermittent fasting can help you balance these hormones, as well as others. For example, fat is very estrogen-rich, so when you lose weight due to timed eating, the relationship between estrogen and progesterone in your body will improve and you'll experience less of the symptoms associated with PMS (Luglio, 2014).

The basis of IF's success lies in the following hormonal processes:

> **Insulin regulation:** Most people hear insulin and think of blood sugar and diabetes. This hormone, however, has many other functions throughout the body, including energy storage (and hence, fat storage), maintaining amino acid levels, and regulating brain functions (Alesio, 2018). So, by managing this hormone, you can impact your health on various levels.

> **Increased human growth hormone (HGH) levels:** Fasting increases the level of this hormone dramatically (Shea et al., 2015). That's exactly what you want to hear if staying young for longer is your aim. I'd go as far as saying that this hormone is one of the most important hormones in the

body since it regulates the lifecycle of the cells in your body. HGH is also responsible for burning fat into energy.

➢ **Cellular repair:** Another fascinating benefit of IF is that it triggers a process called autophagy (Glick, Barth, & Macleod, 2010). Think of it as a housekeeping mechanism where all the damaged parts of cells get eliminated, making space for healing to occur thanks to, you guessed it, HGH (Fung, 2016). To activate this process, your body needs to be deprived of nutrients for a while. The drop in insulin while you're fasting ups the level of glucagon and that stimulates autophagy.

➢ **Gene expression:** Who would've thought that not eating for a few hours a day could cause changes to your genes? It's unbelievable to fathom that something so simple can make such a drastic difference. One study on rodents found that restricting food to a feeding cycle improved metabolic profiles and reduced the risk of obesity and related ailments, such as diabetes, non-alcoholic fatty liver disease, and cancer (Patterson & Sears, 2017). Although data from human studies are limited, the evidence that is available corroborates these findings (Altman & Rathwell, 2009).

Now that you know the driving forces behind IF, let's look at some of the advantages when everything works together.

You Lose Weight

At its root, weight loss is about eating enough to fuel your body and no more. If we remove all the other aspects that impact our weight, like genetics, hormones, and psychology, maintaining, gaining, and losing weight comes down to calories in versus calories out.

When you fast, you have a limited time to eat. Depending on which protocol you choose, you may have a feeding window as small as one hour. If you focus on eating healthy, wholesome foods during this time, it is unlikely that you'll be able to meet your calorie needs for the day. This means you'll be in a caloric deficit, which will lead to weight loss.

Add to that the lower insulin levels and higher HGH levels, and your body basically turns into a fat-burning machine as you fast. One study found that IF can cause weight loss of between three and eight percent in anything from 3–24 weeks (Barnosky et al., 2014). That is a remarkable number. Participants in the same study also lost between four and seven percent of their waist circumference. This shows that IF has the ability to get rid of your stubborn belly fat or visceral fat—the kind of fat known to cause heart disease among other ailments (Chiba et al., 2007).

Earlier, I mentioned how diets can cause muscle loss. That is not something you should worry about when you follow a time-restricted eating program. Research has shown that IF causes less muscle loss than the typical calorie restriction diets out there due to the boost of HGH (Varady, 2011).

Reduces Insulin Resistance

IF can reduce your blood sugar by as much as six percent over the course of 8–12 weeks (Barnosky et al., 2014). Blood sugar drops by an impressive 20–31 percent. Since high blood sugar is the driver of insulin resistance, lowering your blood sugar is vital if you want to normalize your insulin levels. If you don't, you're at risk of getting type 2 diabetes. Regrettably, 11.3% of the U.S. population has been diagnosed with type 2 diabetes (CDC, 2019). This isn't surprising considering that the standard American diet is based on refined carbohydrates and sugars.

Reduces Oxidative Stress and Inflammation

Oxidative stress happens when there's an imbalance between antioxidants and unstable molecules called free radicals. These molecules react with protein, DNA, and other important molecules and damage them—this plays a major role in aging and disease (Pizzino et al., 2017). Through autophagy, oxidation can be reduced, and mitochondrial functionality of cells enhanced (Ahmed et al., 2018).

IF also helps fight inflammation you may not even know you have. Let's face it, society lives on excess—of everything. The problem is that prolonged caloric excess causes systemic low-grade chronic inflammation, which contributes to numerous diseases (Jordan et al., 2019).

Benefits Your Heart

Around 16% of global deaths are caused by heart disease; it is the biggest killer in the world (WHO, 2019). There are many health markers or risk factors that increase a person's risk of heart disease. Some of these are:

- high blood sugar level
- high blood pressure
- high triglycerides
- high cholesterol, especially the bad kind (LDL)
- inflammation

Studies found cardiovascular health benefits from intermittent fasting too (Dong et al., 2020). Although the exact mechanism isn't yet known, the positive impact IF has on heart disease risk factors, such as obesity, diabetes, hypertension, and inflammation cannot be denied. IF is also associated with better recovery after cardiac events.

Helps Prevent Cancer

As explained earlier, the process of autophagy involves breaking down cells and absorbing the broken and dysfunctional parts, chiefly proteins, that build up over time (Bagherniya et al., 2018). This metabolism of unhealthy parts of cells may provide protection against cancer and other degenerative diseases (Amaravadi, Kimmelman, & Debnath, 2019).

Is Good for Your Brain

Although human studies are limited on IF's link to brain health, time-restricted eating sparks the growth of nerve cells in mice and rats (Baik et al., 2020). But the anecdotal evidence showing an increase in alertness levels, as well as improved memory may be enough reason to give it a go.

Then there's the fact that fasting increases brain-derived neurotrophic factor (BDNF)—a protein that keeps you energetic, smart, and happy (Mattson et al., 2018). BDNF not only helps your neurons resist age-related brain diseases such as Alzheimer's, Parkinson's, and Huntington's, but also is a key player in stroke rehabilitation (Conway & Engels, 2020).

Prolongs Your Life

This is what excites me about intermittent fasting the most: The fountain of youth lies in what we eat and when!

IF has been shown to increase the lifespan of fruit flies and rodents. The results of one study are quite dramatic, as rats that ate only every other day lived 83% longer than their non-fasting counterparts (Goodrick et al., 1982).

Further research also found that daily fasting can delay the onset of certain diseases, chiefly fatty liver disease and hepatocellular carcinoma, which are common in aging mice (Mitchell et al., 2019).

Although these are animal studies, considering the known benefits of IF, it makes sense that IF could prolong your life too.

The bottom line is that IF is popular for a reason. The benefits of time-restricted eating go beyond weight loss; it can help you live a longer and healthier life. Another aspect that contributes to IF's attractiveness is the versatility it offers. There are many methods of intermittent fasting you can choose from to help you succeed.

Intermittent Fasting Protocols

The term "intermittent fasting" incorporates any method where you eat only during a specific window of time.

The five most common intermittent fasting approaches are as follows:

1. The 16/8 protocol is popular, especially among those who are dipping their toes into time-restricted eating. The fast is long enough for the benefits of IF to kick in but not long enough to make you feel famished. This fasting method is usually timed in such a way that a big chunk of the actual fast happens when You're sleeping. In fact, it's basically just skipping breakfast. For example, if you eat your last meal at 7 p.m. and you fast for the required 16 hours, your eating window will start at 11 a.m.—just in time to enjoy a delicious lunch. Even though 16/8 is the most

widespread method used, you can adapt it. I always recommend my patients start with 16/8 and once they feel comfortable fasting for 16 hours, they can prolong their fast for 18 hours, then 20, even 24 hours if they feel up to it. There are many people who successfully practice one meal a day (OMAD), on a daily basis.

2. The 5:2 diet is a much milder form of IF. You can eat normally for five days of the week, but then must restrict your calorie intake to 500 on the other two days.

3. Eat-Stop-Eat is where you fast for 24 hours twice a week. How you spread your fasts out is totally up to you and depends on your social life and routine.

4. Alternate-day fasting is when you fast every second day.

5. The Warrior Diet is often confused with OMAD, but there is a slight difference. On the Warrior Diet, you're allowed to snack on raw fruits and veggies throughout the day and then enjoy your large meal at night. OMAD, on the other hand, limits your calorie intake to one meal a day. You're allowed to enjoy tea and coffee without sugar or milk, and water, but nothing else until you sit down for dinner.

Where to Start

Many popular weight-loss regimes require you to weigh your food, limit carbohydrates, avoid fat, and other bothersome and restrictive demands. Another advantage of IF is that if you generally follow a healthy diet focused on wholesome foods, you can go on eating as is just for a limited time.

That being said, fasting is still a lifestyle change and will need some planning.

Here are five tips to increase your likelihood of success.

1. Start Slow

You may feel tempted to try OMAD or the 20/4 protocol. That is admirable and kudos on being so motivated, but unfortunately sudden and dramatic changes to your eating habits usually don't last long. It can be quite jarring to go from eating three square meals a day with snacks in between to only eating once a day. I recommend you start with the 16/8 protocol. If you find that too difficult, try 14/10 until you feel comfortable extending your fast. You can build up to longer fasts if you do it at a steady pace.

One of my former patients increased her fast by 30 minutes every two days and then went 18 hours without eating.

2. Up Your Protein, Fat, and Fiber Intake

Yes, you read that right: Up your fat intake. I know that goes against what you've heard and may even be the opposite of what your health care professional has told you, but hear me out. There are different kinds of fat. I'm not suggesting you stock up on trans or saturated fats found in man-made, highly processed foods. Instead, I want you to eat foods high in monounsaturated and polyunsaturated fats.

Some good fat foods include avocado, nuts, fatty fish, dark chocolate, whole eggs, and chia seeds.

Not only are these fats good for you, but they also make you feel satiated for longer since they are considered calorie dense. Of course, the fact that they're high in calories means you'll have to keep an eye on how much you eat.

Protein and fiber also help you feel fuller for longer and it will keep your blood sugar stable during your fast.

3. Don't Worry About Setbacks

You're only human and there will be days when you find it impossible to fast and end up consuming calories outside of your eating window. That's normal, especially considering the social nature of humans and that many of our celebratory occasions happen around food. Don't be too hard on yourself. If you do have a setback, don't quit; instead, use it as an opportunity to get back on track with even more drive. Remember, IF isn't a diet, so don't treat it like one. It's a versatile eating program you can adapt to fit your life and that includes breaking your fast earlier at times to be able to attend a dinner with family or friends, for example.

4. Exercise in Moderation

In the next chapter, I will deal more extensively with exercise, but when it comes to IF and getting active, easy does it is the way to go. I know you may be tempted to start everything at once to see results faster, but again, if this is your train of thought, you're approaching these changes as a short-term affair and not a new way of life.

Starting a vigorous exercise routine along with IF is going to make it much more difficult to stick to your fast. You're going to get hungry sooner since your body is depleting its glucagon stores while You're hitting the gym. To avoid this increased hunger, slowly increase your activity level until you can exercise at the intensity you want while coping with the accompanying hunger pangs.

5. Plan What to Eat

If you want to maximize the health benefits of intermittent fasting, you must think about what you eat. Wholesome, nutritious foods should win every time. I realize that it isn't always possible with the busy lives we all lead, and at times, the convenience of takeout is just too tempting. Again, if that does happen, take a breath. If you stay on the wagon, for the most part, falling off every now and again won't wipe out all the positive changes in your body.

I find it is much easier to stick to the plan when you actually have one. A shopping list can be your salvation when you're in the grocery store. You don't have to wander aimlessly through the aisles, looking for something to eat. Instead, you can approach it as a mission: Go in, find what you're looking for, go out. No time to notice a new brand of cookies on the shelves.

Another tip I have is to stick to the outer limits of the grocery store. That is usually where all the fresh foods are packed; the processed, sugary foods are usually in the middle.

As long as you eat a balanced diet the majority of the time, you're doing just fine. Avoid overly processed packaged foods like cookies, chips, deep-fried foods, frozen microwaveable meals, etc. Sugar should also be limited as much as you can.

Since what you eat is vital to your overall well-being, I think it's a good idea to take a closer look at the foods you should have on your plate daily.

Enjoy a Balanced Diet

A healthy diet includes eating a variety of foods from the five food groups:

- ➤ vegetables
- ➤ fruits
- ➤ grains
- ➤ protein
- ➤ dairy

When you eat enough of all of the above, you're giving your body the vitamins and minerals it needs to maintain good health and fight against diseases. You also have to keep your calories in mind because, as they say, even a good thing can become a bad thing when done in excess. In other words, if you eat too much even if it is healthy food, it's not good for you.

The USDA recommends that half a person's plate be filled with fruits and vegetables—the bigger the variety the better. The other half should be made up of grains and protein (USDA, 2020). Together with your meal, they also suggest enjoying a serving of dairy.

But before we take a more in-depth look at what you should eat, let's tackle the issue of how much you should eat.

I've mentioned calories quite a few times already and some of you may be wondering what exactly it is. In essence, calories are energy. The food you eat contains a specific amount of stored calories, which are then transformed into energy for breathing, thinking, walking, and all other bodily functions.

For example, men tend to need more energy; similarly, people who are very active require more calories than their sedentary counterparts. As you age, your energy needs change and you may have to recalculate your recommended daily calories on a regular basis. So, keep a close eye on how your body changes and adjust your calories accordingly.

There are numerous calorie calculators online, but if You're unsure, your doctor will be able to help you figure out your energy expenditure.

Fruits

Fruits contain a lot of sugar, and you should enjoy them in moderation. Although it is natural sugar, and it is better than candy, they still affect your blood sugar and can contribute to insulin resistance when consumed in excess.

If you're afraid of consuming too much sugar, you can always stick to low-sugar fruits such as raspberries, strawberries, blackberries, kiwi, grapefruit, watermelon, cantaloupe, and oranges.

The fiber and other nutrients also make fruit a healthier choice than chocolate. It should definitely be your first choice when you want to pacify your sweet tooth. I like to incorporate fruits as a dessert. If you decide not to follow an intermittent fasting protocol, you can also use fruit as a snack between meals.

A top tip is to always select fruits that are in season as they contain the most nutrients.

Vegetables

Vegetables are key to a healthy meal. They contain many essential vitamins, minerals, and antioxidants. I used to tell my patients their plate should look like a rainbow—the wider the variety the larger the range of nutrients.

Colorful vegetables signal the presence of phytochemicals and phytonutrients, which come with a slew of health benefits, chiefly, heart health (Bondonno, 2019).

Grains

Most of the baked goods on the shelves contain refined white flour. That's unfavorable since it has been stripped of most of its nutritional value in the refining process. We end up eating a lot of empty calories when we reach for products made from processed flour.

Whole grain, on the other hand, contains the grain in its entirety, which means the vitamins, minerals, and fiber are still intact. The taste is also more flavorsome.

It's not always easy to switch to whole grain bread, pasta, and baked goods since the available options are somewhat limited when compared to white flour products. At least half of the grains you eat should be whole grains (if you can, shoot for more). Whole grains you can choose from include quinoa, brown rice, barley, oats, and buckwheat.

Protein

Protein is essential for muscle maintenance and development, wound healing, and other important bodily functions. Meat and beans are the two main sources of protein.

Animal-based options like poultry, red meat, and fish are all healthy protein sources. That being said, red meat contains more unhealthy fats than poultry and fish, so I recommend limiting eating beef, mutton, and pork to once a week or less.

Processed meats should be avoided as much as you can since they contain added preservatives and salt, which is bad for your health. Furthermore, processed meats may increase your risk of cancer and other diseases (Battaglia et al., 2015).

Plant-based protein comes from nuts, beans, and soy. Some of the best examples include lentils, beans, peas, sunflower seeds, almonds, and walnuts.

Tofu and tempeh are the most well-known soy-based protein sources.

Soy products have been touted as a wonder 'cure' for menopause as it mimics estrogen in the human body. So, since your natural estrogen levels fluctuate during this time, it is suggested that soy products can manage this change and lessen the symptoms associated with menopause. Think of it as a natural form of estrogen therapy. In fact, there has been a sharp decline in estrogen therapy as women take the natural route.

That being said, I have to mention that the link between soy intake and breast cancer has been investigated for many, many years. Unfortunately, the results aren't conclusive. Some studies found that soy increases cancer risk in high-risk women but reduces the risk in women who start to eat soy products early in life (Messina, 2016). More research is needed, but I recommend you have a chat with your doctor. They know your medical history the best and can consider it with the latest research on soy and cancer in mind.

Dairy

Dairy products are a good source of protein, calcium, and vitamin D. It is also high in fat, and you may want to rope your doctor in to help you decide if you should choose reduced-fat dairy options. As I mentioned earlier, fat isn't as bad as we're led to believe; it's the type of fat that's the problem. But, if you are struggling with high cholesterol, your doctor may recommend you limit your fat intake.

For the vegans among my readers, you're welcome to enjoy milk made from flaxseed, soy, almonds and cashews, oats, and coconut. These milks are often fortified with nutrients and calcium, which make them a wonderful alternative. I do recommend you pay close attention to the label as some of them may contain added sugar.

Fats and Oils

Although not part of the five major food groups, fat is an essential component of a healthy diet. It gives your body energy and promotes cell health. But, as we know, too much of a good thing is hardly ever good. Since fat is high in calories, consuming too much can lead to weight gain and other health complications.

If you stick to eating good fats, you lower your risk of cardiovascular disease. However, what is considered good fats differs from one study to another and often changes. For example, in the past, fat was seen as bad no matter what. That has recently changed to "some fats are good," but the division doesn't stop there. Some experts are steadfast in their belief that saturated fat is bad. Period. While others think it is good for you to consume some of this kind of fat to help your body run as it should (Nettleton et al., 2018). This makes recommendations on fats confusing.

The one thing that everyone agrees on is that trans fats should be avoided at all costs. So, to lessen the confusion, I use to tell my patients to enjoy as much of the good fats as they want, keeping their daily calorie allowance in mind, limit their saturated fat intake, and don't come near foods containing trans fats.

In other words:

- Enjoy vegetable oils and fish oils.
- Limit butter, heavy cream, and cheese.
- Avoid processed and premade foods such as cakes, cookies, donuts, pre-packed crumbed chicken, etc.

To recap, eating a balanced diet means including wholesome food from the five major food groups on your plate. Although dietary guidelines change as new information is discovered, the current recommendation is to eat a wide variety of fruits and vegetables with some lean protein.

These foods are loaded with antioxidants, essential nutrients, and healthy fats, and your body will appreciate you making healthy food choices. Now that you know more about a balanced diet, let's look at some foods that work against aging.

Top 10 Age-Busting Foods

Your skin is your largest organ, and it is also the first indicator of a healthy diet. If you eat wholesome food and keep hydrated, your skin will glow. Research has even found that eating fruits and veggies can fight fine lines and improve your complexion (Schagen et al., 2012).

Here is a list of the top 10 anti-aging foods that keep you looking younger from the inside out. After all, there's only so much that face creams, serums, and masks can do!

1. Watercress

Calcium, potassium, phosphorus, manganese, vitamins A, C, K, B1, and B2. Need I say more? This flavorful green is jammed-packed with vitamins and minerals. Watercress increases blood circulation, which means your skin cells will get enough oxygen to run all the processes that heal and fight aging (Gill et al., 2007). Furthermore, vitamins A and C are known antioxidants that can fight off those harmful free radicals that lead to wrinkles (Zeb, 2015).

Not sure how to enjoy watercress? It is a wonderful addition to any salad as it adds crunch and flavor. You can also enjoy it as a snack between meals.

2. Red bell pepper

As we know, antioxidants are one of the magic bullets against aging. Loaded with antioxidants, red bell pepper is a true powerhouse vegetable. It gets its color from carotenoids, a powerful antioxidant known for its anti-inflammatory properties (Fiedor & Burda, 2014). This protects the skin from pollution, environmental toxins, and sun damage (Stahl & Sies, 2012). On top of that, red bell peppers contain vitamin C, which is great for collagen production.

Make red bell pepper part of your diet as a snack. It's delicious when dipped in hummus—a superfood in its own right.

3. Papaya

Papaya contains an enzyme called papain—one of nature's best anti-inflammatories. By now we know that eating foods high in anti-inflammatory properties combat inflammation caused by free radicals and such, but it can also improve skin elasticity (Mohamed, 2012).

When you enjoy a plate of papaya, you can expect to get a good helping of vitamins A, B, C, K, and E, as well as calcium, potassium, phosphorus, and magnesium.

You can make papaya part of breakfast and enjoy it with some oats, or slice it into a salad for a nice tropical taste. Don't forget to drizzle some lime juice over for extra zing!

You can also make a face mask by smashing papaya and adding some yogurt. The papain in the papaya is a known exfoliator.

4. Blueberries

Anthocyanin is another age-defying antioxidant and—you guessed it—you can find it in blueberries. Not only does anthocyanin protect against sun damage, pollution, and stress, but it also prevents collagen loss (Skrovankova et al., 2015).

Snack on blueberries throughout the day or make it part of a fruit bowl or smoothie.

5. Broccoli

Packed with vitamins C and K, fiber, folate, lutein, calcium, and a variety of antioxidants, broccoli is an anti-aging miracle.

Enjoy it raw as a snack or grill it in the oven with some cheese. Broccoli is one of the few vegetables that actually release more health benefits when you cook it.

6. Spinach

Not only is spinach packed with vitamin C to help boost collagen production, but it also contains vitamin A, which promotes stronger, healthier hair, and vitamin K, which fights inflammation on a cellular level (Shea et al., 2008).

Spinach is a versatile ingredient in the kitchen. You can sauté it, mix it with banana to make a smoothie, or eat it raw as a salad.

7. Nuts

Vitamin E has many mending properties. It helps skin stay moisturized and protected from damaging UV rays. Almonds and walnuts contain a good helping of vitamin E. They're also loaded with omega-3 fatty acids that strengthen cell membranes and give the skin a natural glow by protecting its oil barrier.

Nuts make a great snack but work just as well sprinkled on top of a salad to add some crunch. Try not to remove the skin, research suggests that 50% of the antioxidants are found in the skin (Ros, 2010).

8. Avocado

Avocados contain essential nutrients such as vitamins A, B, C, E, K, carotenoids, potassium, and healthy fatty acids that prevent the negative effects associated with aging (Dreher & Davenport, 2013).

This fruit makes a great addition to smoothies and salads, but you can also apply it topically to moisturize your skin and reduce redness.

9. Sweet potato

Beta-carotene, the antioxidant that gives sweet potatoes their orange color, is converted into vitamin A in the body and helps restore some of your skin's original beauty. It's also high in vitamin C and E, which keep your complexion radiant by blocking harmful free radicals.

Why not make yourself some sweet potato crisps? Slice them as thin as possible, drizzle lightly with olive oil, and pop them into the oven.

10. Pomegranate seeds

There are many reasons why this fruit has been used as medicine for centuries. It is high in vitamin C and an assortment of potent antioxidants. What's more, it contains punicalagins, a compound that helps preserve collagen, ultimately slowing down signs of aging.

Add pomegranate seeds to a bowl of spinach and walnut to make the ultimate age-busting treat.

They say you are what you eat and that is absolutely true. If you want to look and feel your best, you need to fuel your body with wholesome goodness. The more colorful the selection, the better, as the rich shades are signs of potent anti-aging properties.

By choosing the right foods, you can slow down aging from within. If you add the power of intermittent fasting to a healthy diet, you have the ultimate anti-aging recipe in your hands.

In the coming chapter, we'll look at another important part of staying young and looking good: exercise. I'll share with you what type of exercises are best considering your age and provide some tips and tricks to make it part of your daily life.

Chapter Summary

- ➤ Fad diets don't work; there's no quick fix to losing weight.
- ➤ What and when you eat can slow down the aging process.
- ➤ A diet should be a long-term solution that changes your relationship with food.
- ➤ Time-restricted eating has many health benefits.
- ➤ The 16/8 intermittent fasting protocol is the most popular, but you should choose one that fits your lifestyle.
- ➤ A healthy diet includes protein, vegetables, fruit, grain, and dairy.
- ➤ There are good fats and bad fats. Trans fat should be avoided entirely.
- ➤ Choose foods high in antioxidants and anti-inflammatories for the best anti-aging results.

CHAPTER 3:
PHYSICAL HEALTH

No one will deny that exercise is good for you. It not only keeps you fit, but it also keeps you healthy and young. The benefits of getting active include improving heart and lung health. In fact, exercising from a young age has been proven to delay the onset of 40 chronic conditions (Ruegsegger & Booth, 2017). However, it's never too late to start, so don't worry if you haven't exercised your whole life. A study conducted on residents at a nursing home found an increase in activity levels improved their physical and cognitive abilities and had a positive impact on their mental health (Arrieta et al., 2019). Not surprising since exercise is a well-known stress buster and mood booster.

If You're not a fan of exercise, don't feel discouraged. You don't have to spend hours in the gym to reap the anti-aging benefits. Small changes like taking the stairs and not the elevator, walking your dog, or gardening will do—as long as you do it regularly.

In this chapter, I'm going to guide you in doing the right exercises for your age. But first, here's a breakdown of the good that comes from being more physically active.

1. It makes you stronger.

Earlier, I mentioned that losing muscle mass and strength is part of the aging process. This process is called sarcopenia. There are numerous studies that show that resistance training can help slow this process and help you retain your strength. With stronger muscles, everyday activities are easier. Climbing stairs, pushing a heavy door open, cleaning, and opening jars all require a fair amount of strength.

I know you may be concerned that resistance training is too strenuous, and you may be afraid of hurting yourself. Well, researchers found that rates of injuries are similar across all ages and intensities, so it is entirely safe for older adults (Lavin et al., 2019).

2. It improves bone density.

As you get older, your risk of developing osteoporosis increases. Almost half of all adults over 50 are in danger of breaking a bone due to this skeletal disorder (National Osteoporosis Foundation, 2015). Women are more at risk, making it so much more important for you to get physically active. Walking or another aerobic activity, especially after menopause is a must. You won't be able to regain bone mass, but physical activity will prevent any further loss.

Lower impact activities like swimming are a great form of exercise, but not intense enough to affect bone loss. To have a real impact on your bone health, you need to get your heart pumping. Weight-bearing exercises are the most effective. I recommend you also join a yoga or Pilates class to improve your balance to avoid any nasty falls.

3. It keeps your cells young.

Remember the caps on the ends of your cells called telomeres? Exercise can help lengthen them, which will make it possible for your cells to continue dividing and regenerating (Arsenis et al., 2017). This is a surefire way to reduce the risk of age-related diseases.

4. It improves cognitive ability.

Cognitive decline is a reality as you grow older. Your mind won't stay as sharp as it used to be. Physical activity shows a lot of promise in slowing down this deterioration (Erickson et al., 2018). This is partly due to the production of myokines in your muscles when you exercise. These small molecules are beneficial to your brain in many ways.

We don't know everything there is to know about exercise and aging… yet! But one thing we do know is that 30 minutes of light exercise daily is better than no physical activity at all.

Here are some other guidelines when it comes to exercise when you're over 50:

➢ To get the most out of moderate exercise, you should aim for between two and a half hours and five hours a week. If you up the intensity, you can exercise for a total of one hour and fifteen minutes and two and a half hours spread throughout the week.

➢ Muscle-strengthening activities that involve all the major muscle groups should be done twice or more a week, with aerobic exercise being spread evenly throughout. Balance training should be incorporated into your exercise program as many times as possible.

➢ Determine the level of your effort relative to your level of fitness.

➢ If you have a chronic condition, research how your condition affects your ability to be physically active, if at all.

➢ If you struggle to exercise for the minimum recommended time due to a chronic condition or illness, try to be as physically active as you can.

Recommended Activities

Many troubles of aging are due to leading an inactive lifestyle. Our bodies become stiff, we lose muscle mass, our bones turn brittle, and so on. Many of these negative aspects of growing older can be delayed or prevented by regular exercise.

Before you take on any exercise regime, check with your doctor. If you're at risk of heart disease, then you may need to avoid certain activities. Your doctor will be able to guide you in that aspect.

To create a complete fitness program, you can start by choosing an aerobic exercise that you like. You can jog, swim, walk, or even take up a dancing class if you're adventurous enough. Anything that gets your heart pumping can be seen as aerobic exercise. To make sure that you're not pushing yourself too much, try the "talk test"—if you're too out of breath to utter a sentence, then slow down a little.

Next, your exercise program should include resistance and strength training. Not only do these exercises improve your strength and posture, but it also helps slow down bone loss.

I'm a great fan of strength training because you can do it in the comfort of your own home while using your body weight. There's no need to waste money on expensive equipment; all you need is your body, a chair, and optional hand weights.

Here are three of the top strength training exercises that will target your whole body:

1. The Plank

The plank pose is a super exercise. It looks deceptively easy, but you're guaranteed to feel the burn. This exercise targets your core muscles (abdominal and lower back muscles), but that doesn't mean you won't feel it in your arms and legs too. The plank also improves your balance and posture.

There is an easy or a hard way to do a plank. If you're a beginner, lie down on your stomach. Now, bend your arms at the elbow, and push your whole body off the ground as if You're doing a push-up. Hold it there for as long as you can. Make sure your back is straight—your belly button should not be closer to the ground than the rest of your body.

If you're in the mood for more of a challenge, instead of supporting your weight on your forearms, straighten your arms, shifting the support to your hands. This is called a high plank.

The aim is to form a straight line parallel to the ground for as long as you can.

2. Squats

Squats are easy to do at home and it's a great way to help tone your lower body.

If you're totally new to this exercise, use a chair as your guide. Stand in front of it as if you want to have a seat. Lower yourself but stop before touching the seat. Stand back up and repeat multiple times. If you find that you're losing your balance, extend your arms out in front of you.

As you get better at this exercise, you can remove the chair and attempt a deeper squat.

3. Chest Fly

Women have weak chest muscles, and this can negatively impact your posture as you age. The chest fly exercise is a good way to strengthen these muscles.

If you have a pair of hand weights, grab them. If not, then go raid your pantry for two cans that you can grip tightly. Armed with your weights, lie on the floor flat on your back. Your knees should be bent and your feet hip-width apart flat on the ground. With a weight in each hand, open your arms to the side and lower down toward the floor as far as you can. Don't touch the ground, but hover just above it for a few seconds before slowly bringing your hands together above your chest. Repeat. Always keep your elbows slightly bent to prevent locking them out and injuring yourself.

When you're done with your exercise, whether it was aerobics or strength training, you need to stretch. I'd even go as far as saying you should stretch daily, and sometimes, more than once a day! Stretching is a great way to stay flexible and maintain your mobility.

You can join a yoga class, take up Pilates, or just get down on the floor at your home.

Here are some stretching exercises I want to share with you. After doing them, your muscles will feel relaxed, and you'll move around with fewer aches and pains. The only thing you need to remember when you stretch is not to overdo it. If you feel pain, don't hold the stretch. The pain is your body's way of telling you that You're stretching too far and should ease up a little. Although stretching some parts may be more challenging than others, it shouldn't hurt.

Arm opener: Stand with your feet hip-width apart and flat on the floor. Interlace your hands behind your tailbone. Your knuckles should point down. Gently start to push your arms away from your body as far as you can. When you feel a nice stretch, stop, and take a few deep breaths.

Chin drop: Bend your arms in front of you, palms up, pinkies touching. Move your head towards your hands until your palms are on top of your head. Gently let the weight of your arms guide your head as you drop your chin down. When you feel a deep stretch in your neck and shoulders, take a few deep breaths and relax your upper back as you exhale. This will help release tight areas and unnecessary tension.

Hip stretch: Stand and put your feet together. Start to bend forward from your waist slowly. Move your hands down your legs as low as you can. Once you find a comfortable position, bend one knee, then the other while keeping your feet flat. Keep a static stretch for 15 seconds, but if you find one side is tighter, stay there a little longer. Your head should be relaxed, hanging down freely.

Triceps stretch: Plant yourself solidly on the ground—feet hip-width apart. Roll your shoulders back and down. Lift your right arm and reach for the ceiling. Your shoulders should stay down and away from your ears. Bend your right elbow and place your right hand, palm flat, close to the middle of your shoulder blades. Take your left hand and place it on your right arm just above your elbow. You should feel a nice stretch. Hold the position for 15 to 30 seconds and repeat three to five times.

Side-to-side stretch: Your feet should be shoulder-width apart and your toes angled outward. Interlace your fingers and bring your hands up to your chest with palms facing away. Your elbows should point out to either side. Don't move your lower body as you twist your upper body right and left. Keep your head strong and in line with your body. To avoid getting dizzy, gaze forward. Do this 15 times.

Make Exercise Part of Your Daily Life

A healthy lifestyle can't only happen on days when you feel like it—you have to put in the effort to eat correctly and get active daily.

Many women struggle to make exercise part of their daily routine because they have a million things to do. Finding time to get physically active in between school drop-offs and pickup, cleaning, cooking, and working is a difficult task. That's one of the positives of reaching the 50+ mark; your kids have probably flown the nest, freeing up more time to do things for yourself.

If you still find it difficult to incorporate exercise into your day, here are some tips to make physical activity a part of your routine in a sustainable manner.

1. Do Something You Enjoy

If you've spent your whole life sedentary, it is going to take time to get used to the idea of exercise. To speed up the process, it helps you if you choose activities you like. If you absolutely hate walking on a treadmill because you find it boring, don't include it in your fitness program.

If you can't think of any exercises you would like to do, then you must change your thinking. There are many options out there; you just have to do some research and try the ones with the most appeal. Still, there's the chance that you won't like it right away, but exercise requires commitment, so instead of giving up every time you don't like what you have to do, push through.

The best plan is to be open-minded and try the things that spark even just a little interest.

2. Do What You Can

I remember I once had a patient who wore a shirt with a slogan that read, "Tears are just your fat crying." I found it very amusing and even though breaking a sweat was what she was aiming for, she was having a hard time maintaining the pace she started with. For some reason, people tend to think the harder they push themselves, the more impressive the results. The reality is that even the smallest exercise when done regularly can be effective.

You don't even have to join the gym. A brisk walk, clearing out weeds in the garden, and playing ball with your dog all qualify as exercise.

If you attempt to do everything you can think of, not only do you open yourself up for injury, but you increase the likelihood of you throwing in the towel. I recommend you start with 30 minutes a day. You can increase how long you exercise and the types of exercises you do as you go. Use your body and fitness level to guide you.

3. Drop the Excuses

You won't be in the mood to exercise every day. Some days, you may come up with some very innovative excuses not to get moving. The problem is, if you fall for these excuses once, it will become easier to fall for them again, and before you know it, you're back to leading a sedentary life.

Discipline is key to successfully making physical activity a part of your life, but it doesn't come naturally; you have to build it over time. I like to link my discipline levels to my muscles: As my muscles grow, so does my discipline and vice versa.

If you exercise when you don't feel like it, you will turn it into a habit and before you know it, you won't be able to live without being active.

On the days that you find yourself dreaming up excuses, compromise a little. Instead of doing your normal exercise routine, settle on doing only 5–10 minutes. It's the starting part that is the hardest; once you're doing it, you may be surprised that you end up exercising longer.

4. Don't Compare Yourself to Others

Your path is uniquely your own, and so is your body. There are stronger people than you, or people who are better at physical activity. If you compare yourself to them, your confidence may fall, and you may feel like giving up entirely.

Instead of looking outward, look inward. What are the things that you've accomplished? List them no matter how small and then focus on them when you feel you're not good enough.

There's nothing wrong with looking to others for inspiration. The problem comes when you set unrealistic expectations based on what they've achieved. If you can't meet those expectations, your motivation will diminish.

5. Aim for Convenience

It's much easier to stick to your workout routine if it is convenient. If you join a gym that is an hour's drive away from your home, the likelihood of you going is pretty small. When the gym is just up the road, it's much harder to find an excuse not to go.

You should do what you can to set yourself up for success. I have a friend who places her yoga mat within eyesight when she goes to bed. That way, when she wakes up, it is one of the first things she sees, and she can unroll it and start her morning yoga routine.

The main thing to remember is that exercise should be enjoyable for you to make it part of your daily routine. Luckily, there are so many exercises and even "non-exercise exercises" to choose from.

Here are some effortless ways that don't strictly count as exercise but are just as effective:

- ➤ Take your dog for a walk every day.
- ➤ Don't press that elevator button! Instead, use the stairs.
- ➤ Instead of sending emails, walk over to your co-workers and talk to them.
- ➤ Walk at a brisk pace whenever you can to get your heart pumping.
- ➤ Take up a sport, activity, or game you like. If it is something you enjoy, the chances of you sticking to it increase.

All you need to begin is the will to experiment and then the discipline and motivation to follow through.

So far, we've covered how to fuel and move your body. Another important facet of aging well is getting a good night's rest.

Unfortunately, as you age, especially when going through menopause, sleep isn't a constant. In the next chapter, we'll tackle some of the most common sleep problems, as well as ways in which you can overcome them.

Chapter Summary

➤ Exercise has many anti-aging benefits.

➤ Physical activity doesn't need to consume your life. As little as 30 minutes of moderate exercise will improve your body and mind.

➤ Muscle training, aerobic exercise, and stretching are three important components to any exercise regime when You're over 50.

➤ Strength training and stretching will improve your balance.

➤ It's never too late to start exercising.

➤ For exercise to be effective, you have to do it regularly.

➤ Small changes like taking the stairs instead of the elevator is one way to incorporate physical activity into your daily routine.

CHAPTER 4:
SWEET DREAMS

You may have noticed the lines of your forehead forming permanent creases and your skin losing its youthful luster. But what you don't see is that your body is aging on the inside too. When you don't sleep well, this aging process just happens so much faster—a single night's bad rest can make your cells age quicker (American Academy of Sleep Medicine, 2015).

This is significant in our search for prolonged existence. Since sleepless nights can bring about various diseases, it is vital that we find ways to improve our sleeping habits. But what is considered a good night's sleep? Well, the American Academy of Sleep Medicine, recommends a solid seven hours of sleep for older adults. However, it's not only about the hours of sleep you get, but the quality of sleep.

In this chapter, we'll look at how you can improve your sleep in every way possible. But before we learn more about the how, I think it's important to look at all the reasons why you should do what you can to sleep better.

The Importance of Sleep

I gave you an overall reason why sleep is good for you: it is beneficial to your cells, which makes it favorable in the aging process. But I think we have to break it down a little further to investigate the value of sleep more thoroughly.

Considering that up to 35% of adults in the U.S. don't get enough sleep, there's clearly not enough focus on the importance of this daily activity (CDC, 2017).

Here are some of the ways a healthy sleep routine can benefit your body.

Helps You Lose Weight

Not many people know that there is a correlation between sleep and weight. Research has shown that people who sleep fewer than seven hours per night have an increased risk of gaining weight (Brum et al., 2020). In truth, the numbers are dire. Adults who don't get seven hours of sleep are 41% more at risk of becoming obese (Bacaro et al., 2020).

Although there are numerous factors that impact the effect of sleep on weight gain, hormones are one of the main culprits. Ghrelin and leptin are two hormones that trigger our hunger or fullness responses. When we're sleep-deprived, the levels of ghrelin increase, and we feel hungrier; the level of leptin also drops (Ding et al., 2018). This means we won't be able to tell when we're full and we will continue to eat since we won't stop feeling hungry. That's a surefire way to overshoot your daily caloric allowance!

As if that's not enough, people who need sleep lack energy, which may lead to them craving foods packed with sugar and fat to boost their energy intake (Yang, Schnepp, & Tucker, 2019). Combine this with the haywire hunger hormones and You're on a path to a bigger pant size.

Prioritizing sleep is a good way to maintain and even lose weight.

Improves Concentration

When You're tired, your brain is tired. That leads to a loss of concentration and cognition, which negatively impacts your productivity and performance.

Let's look at doctors as an example. We're often overworked, especially during our residency years. One study found that overworked physicians who suffered from moderate, high, and very high sleep deprivation, were up to 97% more likely to make medical errors (Trockel et al., 2020).

On the flip side, getting enough sleep improves academic performance, improves problem-solving skills, and enhances memory (Okano et al., 2019).

Protects Your Heart

One study done with the participation of 19 students found that low sleep quality and duration increases the risk of heart disease by 13% (Krittanawong et al., 2019).

Limited sleep also increases a person's risk of high blood pressure, especially if they already suffer from obstructive sleep apnea (Makarem et al., 2019). For example, people who sleep fewer than five hours, have a 61% higher risk of getting high blood pressure compared to those who slept seven hours or more (Wang et al., 2015).

Lowers Type 2 Diabetes Risk

36 studies with over one million participants had similar findings: short sleep increases your risk of developing type 2 diabetes by 48% (Anothaisintawee et al., 2015).

Since sleep deprivation has such a widespread impact on the body, including decreased insulin sensitivity, increased inflammation, and hunger hormone changes, it is understandable how a person's risk of diabetes increases.

It's Good for Your Mental Health

When it comes to sleep and mental health, you can look at it two ways. On the one hand, those who suffer from depression and anxiety are more likely to struggle to sleep. On the other side, people who haven't been diagnosed with depression or anxiety may develop these disorders due to not being able to sleep.

In both instances, sleep can help maintain good mental health status and improve symptoms of depression and anxiety when they're already present.

It Manages Inflammation

Sleep plays a role in regulating the central nervous system. Chiefly, it forms part of the stress-response systems called the sympathetic nervous system and the hypothalamic-pituitary-adrenal (HPA) axis (Irwin, 2019). That's a mouthful, I know

When you don't sleep enough, inflammatory signaling pathways are activated, which lead to higher levels of inflammation. If this persists, inflammation turns chronic and this can lead to conditions such as heart disease, depression, obesity, type 2 diabetes, Alzheimer's disease, and so on (Irwin, Olmstead & Carrol, 2015).

One thing is clear, taking care of your sleep is one of the ways you take care of your health. In many aspects, it is even more important than nutrition and exercise, yet sadly, it often takes the back seat. If you want to live longer and look better, you must prioritize how many Z's you catch a night. Neglecting this pillar of health may end up erasing the good work you put in eating correctly and exercising.

I don't want to make it sound as if you're making a choice to stay up late and miss out on sleep. I realize there are specific factors that contribute to sleeplessness, especially for women over 50. Let's look at some.

Causes of Sleep Issues

Aging brings with it many changes and one's sleeping pattern doesn't escape unscathed. When we're older, we tend to sleep less deeply than in our younger years. The reasons behind this can vary, but the fact that we tend to develop more health problems that interrupt our sleep is a good example.

The first step to improving your sleeping pattern is to get to the bottom of what is going on. Here are the most common causes of sleep problems. See if you're experiencing one or more of these and then we can address it later.

1. Underlying medical conditions

Secondary sleep problems are often the cause of restless nights. Health ailments such as heart and lung conditions, heartburn, osteoarthritis, urinary problems, depression, anxiety, and neurodegenerative disorders such as Parkinson's or Alzheimer's can disrupt your sleep. You also have to make sure that any medication you're on isn't interfering with your sleep.

If you can pinpoint the underlying problem, you can improve your sleep.

2. Sleep-disordered breathing

Sleep apnea is the most well-known sleep-related breathing disorder (SRBD), of which obstructive sleep apnea (OSA) is the most common form. This is when a person's breathing stops due to an obstruction. As you grow older, the likelihood of developing a SRBD goes up, especially if you're overweight. This is concerning considering that OSA can lead to stroke, heart failure, and coronary artery disease. Thankfully, it is treatable.

3. Restless leg syndrome (RLS)

5–15% of the population meet criteria for RLS, but only less than three percent present severe symptoms (Yep, Walters, & Tsuang, 2012). RLS causes a sensation of crawling, itching, or restlessness in mostly a person's legs when they lie down to sleep. Many of the female patients I had seen who had it described it as maddening. It's not painful, but unpleasant and frustrating. Although the mechanism of RLS isn't entirely understood, it is linked to dopamine and iron levels in the brain.

4. Insomnia

This is the grand-daddy of sleeping issues as between 23–24% of older adults have symptoms of insomnia (Foley et al., 1995). It's important to note that insomnia isn't as simple as struggling to fall asleep for 30 minutes and then drifting off—it is not sleeping, despite having every opportunity to do so, for nights in a row until your daytime functionality decreases.

I think making the distinction between experiencing sleep issues periodically and suffering from insomnia is important if we want to fix the problem. Many people lie awake at night because they're worried about something, for example. That wouldn't be considered insomnia.

If you're not sure if you have insomnia, I recommend you track your sleep. Write down when you go to sleep, when you wake up, how long you slept, if you considered it a good night's rest, etc. A few bad nights scattered in between primarily good nights shouldn't be labeled as insomnia.

Okay, so you're finding it difficult to sleep. Easy fix, no? Just head over to your pharmacy and get some sleeping pills. No, stop! Sedatives should always be seen as the last resort. Most medications that make you sleep are bad for your brain functionality (Kerrison, n.d.). Add to that the fact that benzodiazepines such as Ativan, Xanax, Restoril, and Valium commonly prescribed for sleep disorders are habit-forming.

Instead, let's look at some other proven approaches to improving your sleep.

How to Treat Sleeplessness

If you're looking for professional help to treat your sleep issues, find someone who offers:

Cognitive-behavioral therapy for insomnia (CBT-I): This is a special form of therapy that helps a person deal with negative thought patterns that lead to insomnia. It also teaches you relaxation practices and other behavioral techniques that will improve your sleep.

Brief behavioral treatment of insomnia (BBTI): This is similar to CBT-I but is designed to be delivered in a shorter period. BBTI is known to be especially effective in reducing nighttime urination (Tyagi et al., 2014).

Get a Restful Night's Sleep

I've got some good news: In chapters one and two, we already covered two major factors that will contribute to a good night's rest: mindfulness and exercise. So, you're well on your way to uninterrupted sleep. To help you get there, you can also try the following:

1. Manage the temperature

As soon as you lie down, your body cools down, and when you get up, its temperature rises again. Considering this, you may want to set the thermostat in your room to a cool 60–67°F.

Individual preferences vary, so you will have to find your sweet spot, but generally, a colder temperature works better.

You can also take a warm bath or shower before bed. When your body cools down afterward, it may trigger your brain to go into sleep mode (Romeijn, Raymann, & Most, 2012). It also improves your sleep efficiency and quality.

2. Breathe

The 4–7–8 breathing method is a powerful way to get your body to relax (Legg, 2018). Developed by Dr. Andrew Weil, it is based on breath control techniques employed in yoga. When done correctly, it relaxes the nervous system.

Here's how to do it:

- ➢ Place the tip of your tongue to the roof of your mouth and move it down until you feel your front teeth.
- ➢ With your mouth closed, inhale through your nose and count until four.
- ➢ Hold your breath as you count to seven.
- ➢ Open your mouth and exhale totally as you count to eight.

Repeat four more times or more if you're extra tense.

3. Set a sleep schedule

The human body loves routine. Have you noticed how, after eating at the same time for a few days, you feel your tummy grumbling as a reminder around the same time? In some respects, we can train ourselves to do certain things at specific times.

When it comes to sleep, our bodies come with a built-in regulatory system known as the circadian rhythm. Think of this as an internal clock that signals our body to wake up during the day and fall asleep at night.

If your circadian rhythm is out, which often happens if you have sleeping problems, you can help reset it by going to sleep and waking up at set times. It won't be long before your body has adjusted to this schedule, and you fall asleep with ease and wake up feeling refreshed.

I recommend you incorporate 30 to 40 minutes into your bedtime routine where you can wind down, relax, and prepare your body for sleep.

4. Manage light exposure

This builds on the previous point. In the time just before bed when you are unwinding, avoid bright lights. Light influences circadian rhythm and can make it difficult for you to fall asleep.

During the day, your body is exposed to bright light—both natural and artificial—which is a cue to stay awake. At night, darkness promotes sleepiness. This happens due to a boost in melatonin, a hormone that encourages sleep.

When you watch TV, play games, or spend time scrolling through social media on your phone, you're making it harder for you to fall asleep. Electronic devices radiate blue light, which suppresses melatonin (Gooley et al., 2011).

So, put down your phone or any other electronic devices and avoid any other sources of bright light that can stop you from having a solid seven hours of sleep.

5. Don't look at the clock

I'm sure you've woken up in the middle of the night and glanced over to the clock to see what time it is. One of two things probably happened: You saw that you still had a lot of time to rest and snuggled into your pillow to continue sleeping, or you fret over the fact that you can't fall back asleep and start thinking just how tired you're going to be tomorrow.

You can see how the second scenario is problematic as it causes a lot of anxiety, which triggers other harmful processes in your body. What's worse is when you constantly wake up at night and can't fall back asleep, your body's internal clock may confuse this as your new sleep cycle. As a result, you may wake up every night even though you would've slept through.

6. Avoid daytime naps

When my father was alive, he was a napper. He loved a short afternoon siesta to recharge his batteries. The only problem is that it affected his quality of sleep at night. This led him to feeling sleepy during the day, which meant he had to take a nap, and so a vicious circle started.

Study after study has found that daytime naps lead to poor sleep quality and sleep deprivation (Ye et al., 2015). Frequent napping also leads to more depressive symptoms and limited physical activity in older folks (Hays, Blazer, & Foley, 1996).

That being said, there is some research that shows no correlation between daytime napping and nighttime sleep issues. You'll know best if it affects your sleep negatively or not. If you do find that you lie awake at night after sleeping during the day, try to limit future naps to 30 minutes or less as early in the day as possible.

7. Watch what you eat, and when

There's this belief that eating a high-carb meal will make you enjoy a good night's rest. Although it is true that carbs will make you sleepy and help you fall asleep faster, it doesn't promote restful sleep. If it's a deeper and more peaceful sleep you're after, then reach for the olive oil and drizzle it on generously. High-fat food has been shown to encourage deep sleep (St-Onge, Mikic, & Pietrolungo, 2016).

What's interesting is that it's not the fact that you're eating more calories when you eat fat that is causing the improvement in sleep. If you follow a high-carb/low-fat diet that contains exactly the same number of calories as a low-carb/high-fat diet, you'll still struggle to fall asleep (Lindseth & Murray, 2016).

If you can't go without having a high-carb meal for dinner, try to eat it no less than four hours before bedtime. That gives you enough time to digest it.

8. Turn up the radio

Music can improve sleep disorders such as insomnia (Wang, Sun, & Zang, 2014). Of course, what type of music you listen to matters. Ideally, you should opt for something that is relaxing. Buddhist music is especially powerful as it can make you fall asleep sooner (Lai et al., 2015).

Overall, listening to soothing music for 45 minutes before bedtime increases your chances of having a restful and deeper sleep.

9. Watch what you drink

We all know that caffeine is a stimulant, so it goes without saying that you should avoid drinking coffee or consuming any other food or drink that contains caffeine. Depending on your sensitivity to stimulants, you may want to stop drinking coffee at least six hours before going to bed to increase your chances of falling asleep easily.

Instead of coffee, I recommend you sip on some tea that helps promote relaxation. Chamomile is a solid favorite of mine, while teas that include passionflower and magnolia have also been proven to work (Guerrero & Medina, 2017; Xue et al., 2020). I have friends that are tea lovers, and they have two common go-to recipes to help combat sleeplessness.

Valerian Tea

Valerian root has been used for ages to soothe nerves and relieve anxiety. Other benefits include curing headaches and migraines, promoting mental agility, treating hyperactivity, and promoting good sleep.

To make this tea all you need to do is infuse a teaspoon of valerian root in boiling water for 15 minutes. Pour it through a strainer and enjoy!

Cinnamon Tonic

If you love the taste of cinnamon, then you'll love this brew. Not only is cinnamon a sleep aid, but it is jam-packed with a host of other health benefits including decreasing your risk of heart disease, improving insulin sensitivity, lowering blood sugar levels, and fighting bacterial and fungal infections.

To make this drink, you'll need:

➤ 3 cinnamon sticks (use powder if you don't have sticks)
➤ 1 tablespoon cloves

- ➤ 1 tablespoon all-spice berries
- ➤ 15 bay leaves
- ➤ 2 pieces of fresh ginger cut into pieces
- ➤ ½ teaspoon peppercorns (optional)
- ➤ 10 cups of water

Once you've gathered all your ingredients, combine all ingredients in a large pot and bring to a boil. Reduce the heat to low and let it steep for two to three hours. You can enjoy it hot or cold after straining into a container. Add some honey for sweetness and an extra boost of goodness.

10. Take Supplements

Although sleeping pills and benzodiazepines aren't recommended, nothing is stopping you from using certain supplements to help you fall asleep.

Many of the supplements work by boosting the production of specific sleep-inducing hormones in your brain. That's why it is safe; it's not adding some unnatural element to make you sleep. You also get supplements that work by calming brain activity.

Here are the top ones I suggest you look into:

Magnesium: Drinking 500 mg per day can improve your sleep. It works by activating the neurotransmitters in charge of sleep.

5-Hydroxytryptophan (5-HTP): Serotonin regulations sleep. When you take 5-HTP, you're boosting your serotonin levels, which will help you sleep. You only need to take 600 mg per day to see results.

L-theanine: This amino acid won't help induce sleep, but it will help you relax. A dose of 400 mg per day will have the desired effect.

Melatonin: You've already read about this natural sleep hormone. The ability to take it as a supplement is a wonderful way to regulate your sleep pattern. Take 0.5–5 mg two hours before bedtime and you'll experience a remarkable improvement in sleep.

One thing is certain, sleep is not something you can overlook as you strive to improve your health, and ultimately, your lifespan. Not sleeping enough may seem insignificant to you because it's nothing a nap can't fix. The reality is, although you may not feel it on a cellular level, the lack of sleep is causing your cells to age at an increased rate.

I shared various things you can implement to improve your sleep pattern. What's exciting is that by making a few small adjustments, you won't only feel and look better, but you'll actively prevent many of the age-related diseases that strike fear in your heart. We really have more power than we think we have!

In the next chapter, we're going to look at ways to boost your energy levels, which will make it much easier to apply some of the things you've already read about.

Chapter Summary

> ➤ Losing sleep is causing your body to age on the outside and inside.

> ➤ Too little sleep increases your chance of gaining weight.

> ➤ You're at risk of high blood pressure if you sleep less than five hours a night.

> ➤ Age-related health issues can interrupt your sleep.

> ➤ Sleep medication is bad for your brain; take supplements instead.

> ➤ Stop drinking caffeine six hours before you go to bed and limit carbs during dinner.

CHAPTER 5:
RESTORING YOUR ENERGY

As you continue reading this book, I hope you're starting to see that your body goes through many changes as it ages. It's a normal part of life-one that we should accept to age gracefully.

With all the things happening behind the scenes, you may often feel drained without knowing why. In women, the fall of estrogen during menopause causes extreme tiredness. A reduction in muscle mass, a slower metabolism, and less nutrient absorption also contribute to feeling fatigued.

Alas, this lack of energy leads to a lifestyle that isn't conducive to anti-aging. We're too tired to exercise, cook a healthy meal, meditate, or do anything else that will actually make us feel better. This initiates a vicious cycle; our inability to do things that are good for us causes us not to want to do them anymore. We lose our drive and motivation to live a healthier life because what's the point? We're too tired to *live* anyway!

Before we know it, we're back to leading a sedentary lifestyle and eating food with little to no nutritional value. This leads to us feeling depressed because we're feeling our age, not to mention that we're stressed about the various health concerns that come with life over 50. Sleepless nights, tossing and turning while we dream up worst-case scenarios are inevitable. What is the result? We become a self-fulfilling prophecy: Our age gets the best of us.

The truth is, fighting against the clock is a full-time job. The good news is the more you do it, the easier it gets, and the healthier habits you cultivate, the easier it is to counteract the changes happening in your body. These healthy habits may not cure age-related diseases, but they may decrease your risk factors for getting them and curtail their onset.

I'm a big fan of doing things naturally. I'm thankful that not everything about aging is out of our control. There are steps we can take to feel better as we grow older. It's up to you to make a conscious choice to use the influence you have to improve your life.

Boost Your Energy Naturally

So, how do you get your oomph back? You'll be surprised by how easy it is to feel more energized. All you need to do is make a few small changes and you'll be back to chasing your grandkids around in the garden in no time!

Unsurprisingly, quality sleep, following a nutritious diet, stress reduction, and exercise, are four of the top ways to combat age-related fatigue. Since we already covered why those lifestyle changes are good for you, let's look at other ways to lead an energy-boosting life.

1. Quit smoking

I always tell my patients there's a warning on cigarette packaging for a reason, yet it remains one of the main preventable causes of ill-health and premature death worldwide.

Smoking adversely affects your health in many ways, and it increases your risk of numerous chronic illnesses. But when we look at how it saps your energy, it comes down to what it does to your lungs. Over time, smoking reduces the efficiency of your lungs resulting in a decrease in oxygen in your blood (Tantisuwat & Thaveerathitham, 2014). The result? You feel tired.

2. Go slow on the drinks

Time to bust another myth. Drinking alcohol before bed will not make you fall asleep faster. It actually reduces the quality of your sleep (Park et al., 2015). How? Well, alcohol increases the production of urine, which means you will have to get up to go to the toilet one or more times during the night. So, you'll wake up feeling tired.

Remember, fight the urge to take a nap! You don't want to kick-start a cycle of napping during the day and staying awake at night.

3. Avoid too much sugar

It's true that sugar gives you an energy boost, but the problem is that it only lasts a short while before you're back in your slump. You may even feel worse after the blood sugar spike wears off. Some people report feeling 26% more drained following a diet high in added sugar, compared to when they limited their refined sugar consumption and enjoyed fresh fruits instead (Breymeyer et al., 2016).

4. Stay hydrated

When athletes are dehydrated, they feel tired and their performance drops (Barley et al., 2018). Drinking enough water not only impacts our energy levels, but how our brain functions, and even our mood. This shows just how important it is to stay hydrated. As a woman over 50, you also need to be cognizant of the fact that you won't always feel thirsty when your body needs water. You have to consciously remind yourself to drink throughout the day.

5. Form connections

It's easy to become isolated when you're struggling with growing older. This is largely due to the stigma around aging we covered in chapter 1. You have to fight against detaching from the world. Socializing energizes you and increases your mood. Furthermore, it offers you a form of support.

Aren't you happy that drinking enough water, following a wholesome diet, sleeping enough, exercising, and spending time with friends and family can give you an energy boost to get through your day?

If you're struggling with low energy levels, have a look at your lifestyle and see what you're doing that may be making you tired. While you're doing that, think about your energy levels throughout the day. Are there times when you have more energy and times when you can hardly stay awake? This information can be valuable in planning your days. Let me explain.

Discover Your High-Energy Moments

With the fluctuating energy levels You're going to experience as you grow older, you must work smart with your time if you want to reach your goals. One way to do this is to figure out when you have the most energy during the day. You can then save the important things you have to do for this time.

To discover your energy flow, you have to observe yourself closely. Start by thinking back to the previous section. Are you doing everything you can to increase your energy levels? Be honest with yourself if you want a true reflection of how your energy levels rise and fall.

Next, pay attention to how you feel at certain times during the day. Do you think altering your sleep, exercise, or eating habits can further extend your vitality? If so, make a few tweaks and reassess the following day.

As you continue to observe yourself, you may discover that you experience energy dips at around the same time each day. Similarly, your energy may rise at specific times daily. Maybe You're a morning person ready to take on the world until around 3 p.m. Alternatively, you may only feel energized in the evening after dinner.

You may also notice that your environment affects your energy levels, as do other external factors.

In the end, you want to know when you experience:

High-clarity periods: This is the time of the day when you're able to think clearly. You want to focus on activities that require more brain power. For example, I am completely clear-headed the first hour after waking up. I use this time to plan out my day in a strategic manner to optimize my time. Other people find they think more clearly after lunch. Whatever the case may be, don't let this time of clarity and focus go to waste.

High-energy periods: There will be a time in the day when you want to do everything at once and help out the world while you're at it. This is when your energy is the highest. Your most important tasks should be reserved for high-energy pockets—

you'll get them done well and on time. Of course, your high-energy period may be at 11 p.m., so you will need to adjust your routine to make the most out of your energy patterns.

Low-energy periods: When you struggle to focus and you want nothing more than to get into bed and sleep, then you're experiencing a low-energy period. You won't want to work at this time, and you shouldn't because the work you'll do won't be up to your normal standards. If you can, wait it out—give your body a break and allow it to rest.

Restless periods: It's difficult to get work done when all you want to do is move. Be smart about it; use this time to exercise. It will help you release the restless energy while increasing your overall energy levels. If you have no choice but to work while feeling restless, it's best to do something that doesn't require a lot of focus. For example, clear your emails, return phone calls, or do some filing.

Using this information, you can structure your life around your expected energy levels. Scheduling your workload with your energy patterns in mind can improve the quality of work you produce, as well as increase your overall productivity. What's more, you'll enjoy life because you'll match your energy level with the right tasks and will give your body a break when it signals for one.

Your life doesn't have to end when you turn 50. Yes, there are negative aspects of growing older, but you're not totally powerless. Take the inevitable drop in energy as an example. There are many straightforward and simple changes you can make to your life to overcome lethargy. And you know what else is great? Many of the changes that fill your energy tank also have other anti-aging benefits. So, you end up addressing more than one problem with just a few basic changes.

In the coming chapter, I will focus on common illnesses prevalent in older age. But, considering the mountains of research on how a healthy diet, exercise, sleep, and mindfulness (among other things) reduce your risk of getting numerous age-related diseases, I wouldn't be too worried if I were you.

Chapter Summary

> The reduction of estrogen causes extreme fatigue.

> Lessening muscle mass, a slower metabolism, and less nutrient absorption also play a role in depleting your energy levels.

> Constant fatigue drains you of your motivation to live a healthy lifestyle.

> Not everything about aging is out of your control; you have the power to make changes that will keep you healthy.

> There are many ways to boost your energy levels naturally. Diet, sleep, exercise, and stress reduction are top examples.

> You can schedule your day around your energy levels.

CHAPTER 6:
PREVENTING ILLNESS

strongly believe hitting the big five-o deserves to be celebrated. Your kids have (hopefully) left the home, your investments are starting to mature, you're wiser, and you have more time for yourself, to name only a few of the positives of reaching this milestone.

It's never a good idea to focus only on the negatives, so applaud the fact that you've traveled around the sun 50+ times!

One downside to getting older is that you have to start paying closer attention to your health. Many chronic health conditions start showing up in midlife. Luckily, many of these conditions can be managed; if they're spotted early and treated immediately, you can prevent serious complications.

The seven most common conditions for women over 50 that you need to keep an eye out for are:

1. High Blood Pressure

This is one of the most common conditions I have seen among my more mature patients. One reason why instances of high blood pressure increase in people over 50 are the changes to our vascular system as we age. Arteries lose their elasticity and become stiff, which causes the pressure inside to build.

What makes high blood pressure dangerous is that it isn't always present with symptoms—even when readings are sky-high. When symptoms do appear, it is usually when blood pressure is so high it is considered life-threatening. Although non-specific, symptoms to look out for are headaches, shortness of breath, and nosebleeds.

If you've been diagnosed with high blood pressure, you'll be excited to know that lifestyle plays a key role in managing your blood pressure. In other words, if you've been applying what you've read thus far, you've lowered your blood pressure without even knowing it!

Let's recap the lifestyle changes we've covered so far and look at why it lowers your blood pressure.

Lose weight: When your weight increases, so does your blood pressure. If you lose the excess weight—even a small amount—you'll reduce your blood pressure. For the readers who like figures: It is possible to reduce your blood pressure by about 1 millimeter of mercury (mm Hg) for every 2.2 pounds of weight loss.

Exercise: Two and a half hours of exercise spread throughout the week can lower your blood pressure significantly if you have high blood pressure. However, consistency is key. If you stop exercising suddenly, your blood pressure will shoot up again.

Follow a healthy diet: A wholesome diet consisting of whole grains, fruits, vegetables, and dairy can lower your blood pressure by more than 10 mm Hg. Hypertension has its very own eating plan called the Dietary Approaches to Stop Hypertension (DASH) diet. It places a lot of emphasis on eating foods rich in potassium, magnesium, and calcium, and avoiding foods high in sodium, added sugar, and especially saturated fat. Basically, eating a nutrient-dense, healthy diet free from overly processed foods. Sound familiar? Chapter 2 in a nutshell!

Watch the alcohol: It's recommended that women limit their alcohol consumption to one drink a day. In fact, one drink a day has the potential to lower your blood pressure by four mm Hg. If you overdo it, the positive impact of alcohol on your health is replaced with high blood pressure, inflammation, brain damage, and other consequences that promote aging.

Stop smoking: Your blood pressure spikes after each cigarette you have (Omvik, 1996). When you quit, your blood pressure will revert to normal.

Reduce stress: Even though more research is needed on the link between chronic stress and blood pressure, the fact that there is a link is undeniable. It's more how chronic stress affects blood pressure that needs further investigating, and not if it does contribute to high blood pressure—That's an observable fact. If you suffer from stress, take some time to get to the root of it. Once you know the cause, you can start thinking of ways to reduce it or, better yet, eliminate it.

2. High Cholesterol

Cholesterol is a build-up of fatty deposits inside your blood vessels. For as long as your cholesterol is high, this waxy substance (plaque) will thicken until it slows or blocks blood flow entirely. As if that isn't scary enough, the plaque can break free from the blood vessel wall and cause a blood clot, which can lead to a heart attack or stroke.

You won't know you have high cholesterol unless you get your blood tested.

Although high cholesterol can be inherited, it is more often caused by unhealthy lifestyle choices. If you change these bad habits, you can reduce high cholesterol.

A healthy diet, regular physical activity, decent sleep, and limited stress will present as a golden thread throughout this chapter as lifestyle plays a crucial role in preventing these age-related diseases.

When it comes to high cholesterol, I have some extra weapons against it that you can add to your arsenal.

Eat soluble fiber: Although humans can't digest these compounds, the beneficial bacteria in your gut can! The probiotics in your intestines need soluble fiber for their nutrition, and if they're happy, you'll be happy as they can help reduce LDL—bad cholesterol—levels (Ho et al., 2017).

Some good sources of soluble fiber include:

➢ beans and lentils

➢ brussel sprouts

➢ oat cereals

➢ fruits

➢ flaxseed

➢ peas

Consume plant sterols and stanols: Plants also have cholesterol and when consumed by humans, they're absorbed like cholesterol. The main difference is that plant cholesterol doesn't clog arteries; instead, it competes with human cholesterol and this rivalry ends up reducing human cholesterol levels. You do get some sterols and stanols from vegetable oils, but considering the health benefits of plant cholesterol, it is available in supplement form.

3. Diabetes

Your doctor will most likely screen you for diabetes at the same time that they're checking your cholesterol. People 50 years and older are most at risk of developing type 2 diabetes, so it's good to make sure You're in the clear. Also, since the warning signs are often silent, it's important to test before it goes untreated for too long, which can create dangerous complications such as kidney disease, heart disease, and vision loss.

Some known symptoms of type 2 diabetes include:

➢ frequent urination
➢ increased thirst
➢ unintended weight loss
➢ increased hunger
➢ blurred vision
➢ fatigue
➢ slow healing of broken skin
➢ tingling in the hands and feet

These signs develop slowly and often go undetected. It is entirely possible to live with type 2 diabetes for years without knowing it.

There's no cure for type 2 diabetes, but you can manage it with lifestyle changes.

4. Arthritis

Joint pain and stiffness can start long before middle age, but it typically gets worse after 50. The two most common types of arthritis are rheumatoid arthritis and osteoarthritis. Rheumatoid arthritis is where the immune system attacks the joints in the body. Osteoarthritis is "general wear-and-tear" arthritis, where the tissue that covers the end of the bones at the joint breaks down. Psoriasis, lupus, and some other underlying diseases can also cause various other types of arthritis.

You're at risk of getting arthritis if:

➤ There's a family history of arthritis.

➤ You're 50-plus years old.

➤ You're a woman.

➤ You sustained a joint injury at one time.

➤ You're overweight.

With more than 100 different types of arthritis—each developing differently yet equally painful—it's good to know that healthy habits can reduce the risk of this condition.

Other than the main lifestyle changes, what else can you do to keep arthritis at bay?

Up your omega-3s: This polyunsaturated fat reduces inflammation in the body, including the joints. It is recommended that you eat a 3.5-ounce serving of salmon, trout, mackerel, or sardines twice a week (USDA, n.d.).

For our vegetarian and vegan friends, nuts and seeds, plant oils, fortified juices, and soy beverages are excellent omega-3 sources.

Avoid injury: It's natural for our joints to get worn out over time. If you add an injury on top of the usual wear-and-tear, the cartilage may get damaged, which will lead to rapid deterioration. To avoid injury, make sure you warm up before exercising and use the correct safety equipment to protect yourself.

5. Osteoporosis

Women are at great risk of their bones weakening once they hit 50. Close to 20% of middle-aged and older women in America have osteoporosis (CDC, 2019). This is due to the fact that bone density tends to drop when estrogen production goes down during menopause.

As with most of the diseases on the list so far, there are no noticeable symptoms until it increases in severity. As the osteoporosis progresses and your bones have been weakened, you may experience:

- ➢ back pain
- ➢ loss of height
- ➢ brittle bones that fracture or break easily
- ➢ stooped posture

There are various factors that increase your likelihood of developing osteoporosis. Your age, race, sex, family history, and body frame are considered 'unchangeable' risks.

Your lifestyle choices, on the other hand, are wholly in your control. For example, you can increase your calcium intake and supplement with vitamin D to help slow down bone deterioration. Likewise, you can take up strength training to increase bone mass.

6. Cancer

No one wants to hear they have the big 'C,' but being blind to the reality that you're at high risk because of your age is not favorable to living a long, healthy life. You must get routine screenings in your 50s; a mammogram at least every two years to check for breast cancer, as well as colon cancer screenings even more regularly.

Symptoms of cancer depend on what part of the body it affects, but there are some general symptoms you can look out for, including:

> ➢ fatigue
> ➢ lump or thickening of tissue under the skin
> ➢ unintended weight loss or gain
> ➢ skin darkening, yellowing, or redness, as well as sores that won't heal

➢ changes in bowel habits

➢ trouble breathing

➢ persistent indigestion

➢ unexplained muscle or joint point

The message around cancer prevention is conflicting. You'll find many cancer-prevention tips but just as many studies advising against them. The only thing that is well-accepted across the board is that the likelihood of you developing cancer is affected by your lifestyle choices. All you need to do is take charge and start making healthier choices. Getting screened regularly and eating a healthy diet are only two examples, let's look at some others.

Don't smoke: Smoking puts you on a collision course with the big 'C' as it has been linked to various types of cancer. Even chewing tobacco should be avoided as it can cause cancer of the oral cavity, as well as the pancreas (CDC, 2021).

Use sunscreen: Skin cancer is the most preventable kind of cancer, yet the most common. To protect yourself, use a broad-spectrum SPF-30 sunscreen, even on cloudy days. Reapply every two hours or more if You're sweating or spending time in the water.

Get the jab: Certain viral infections can trigger the development of various cancers. Hepatitis B, for example, can cause liver cancer and human papillomavirus (HPV) can lead to cervical cancer. Both these infections have vaccines as a prevention measure, so talk to your doctor about getting vaccinated if you haven't already. Although it is recommended children get the HPV vaccine at 11 and 12 years, a variant of the vaccine has been approved for adult use as well.

7. Anxiety and Depression

We all dream of peace and quiet in our golden years. The reality, however, is vastly different. Whether it's financial troubles, children, work, or family feuds, there's a big possibility that you're stressed. The strain this stress causes takes a toll on your mental well-being and this will adversely affect your physical health.

One thing has become apparent in our journey to longevity so far. Your weight, blood pressure, cholesterol, cancer risk, and physical health in general, are rooted in behaviors. Those behaviors, in turn, are embedded in your emotional health.

In other words, your emotions impact your behavior (lifestyle choices), which determine your physical well-being. If your mental state isn't at its best, it will trickle down and impact the rest of your being. That is why I always told my patients when I was in practice to give me a holistic view of their symptoms. Are they stressed? Overly emotional? Do they feel depressed?

When a person's leg is hurting, we find the cause and heal it. Yet, when the chemicals in our brains are a little off, we stay quiet and hope for the best. Your brain is an organ too, so what's wrong with treating it like one and addressing mental disorders as you would a broken leg?

I realize that it may be because mental illnesses aren't so obvious; the symptoms aren't visible—we can't put a cast on it or give you crutches to walk with.

For example, symptoms of depression and anxiety include:

➢ feeling sad, tearful, and hopeless
➢ experiencing outbursts of anger and irritability over insignificant matters
➢ loss of interest in things that you once found pleasurable
➢ sleeping too much or difficulty sleeping
➢ lack of energy
➢ reduced appetite or increased cravings

These mood disorders can be triggered by numerous factors, including childhood trauma, stress build-up, your personality, genetics, drug and alcohol abuse, and the presence of other mental health disorders.

Regular exercise, eating a balanced diet, getting enough sleep, and managing stress will help you manage your depression and anxiety and can even lessen their severity. There are also various medications on the market, but first, have a chat with your doctor and get their opinion on what they think you need.

So, now you know what diseases are common during midlife, but I didn't share this information with you to scare you. My goal was to encourage you and inspire you to take control of your health. Being confronted with everything that can go wrong is a rude awakening, but realizing that you have the ability to stop these diseases in their tracks, or at the very least slow them down significantly, should raise your spirits.

You may have made the wrong lifestyle choices in the past, but it is never too late to change how you do things. If you don't, your last years on earth won't be nearly as pleasant as they can be.

In the end, it's all about what you want to achieve. For me, life began at 50. If you want to say the same, you'll have to make it happen! Let's start by teaching you how to make happiness happen.

Chapter Summary

➢ You've traveled around the sun 50 or more times. Celebrate that!

➢ There are many chronic health conditions that show up in midlife.

➢ The most common age-related diseases don't always have clear symptoms.

➢ Controlling your weight, exercising, following a wholesome diet, reducing stress, limiting alcohol, and not smoking are the healthiest lifestyle choices you can make to prevent or manage diseases.

➢ If you're 50 or older, You're at risk of developing type 2 diabetes.

➢ Routine screening is recommended to catch cancer in the early stages.

➢ Your brain is an organ too, so allow your doctor to treat it as one—don't hide symptoms of depression or anxiety.

CHAPTER 7:
FIND HAPPINESS THROUGH GRATITUDE

S o, here you are. You're 50 or older and you've either achieved most of the goals you've been pursuing or you're far from being where you thought you'd be at this age. What if I told you that midlife is a wonderful time to start a new life?

Yes, the prospect of aging isn't attractive; no one wants to see and feel themselves getting older, but by focusing on your health, you create the possibility of living the life you want.

The reality is that people are living longer, and this life expectancy will continue to increase (Oeppen, 2002). Considering this, what if you lived to be 100 or older while maintaining good health? That gives you around another 50 years to live!

Take a bit of time to let that sink in. Fifty extra years to live but with one major difference: You're not starting from scratch but continuing with financial security (hopefully), experience, and wisdom.

You can do so many things; your mindset is your only obstacle. If you think life is over at 50, then, for you, it will be.

Life Starts at 50

When you're younger, the search for happiness can often feel like grasping at thin air. If you ask me, that's because we're somewhat all over the place early on. We want to do everything and end up doing very little. Happiness means going out clubbing with friends one day; the next day, happiness is buying a new TV.

Although there is nothing wrong with finding joy in the small things in life, it's sometimes hard to see the bigger picture when you're young. However, as you age and gain wisdom, your definition of happiness changes—it's not so much about collecting 'things' anymore, but more about leading an authentic existence.

If you're not sure yet what makes you happy, there are some things you can do that will increase your happiness without you realizing it until you sit back with a smile on your face thinking how content you are.

Take Care of Your Basic Needs

You won't feel like doing any fun things on this list if you're not in the right mood. As we know, many factors impact how we feel. In order to set yourself up for success, you need to build your happiness on a foundation of a healthy diet, exercise, restful sleep, and other healthy lifestyle choices. When you fuel your body the right way and give it time to recharge, you'll have the energy and the right attitude to work toward becoming happier.

When you realize your mood is low, investigate why. Ask yourself if:

➢ you slept enough
➢ you've been eating nutritiously lately
➢ you drank enough water
➢ you exercise or were physically active in some way

Have you ever heard of the term 'hangry'? That's when you're so hungry, you're angry. That's a good example of how your body and mind impact each other. In this case, all you need to do is eat something and your mood will lift. A simple way to increase your happiness!

Chanel Your Creative Self

Creativity is a wonderful mood-booster; it can even help alleviate the symptoms of depression ("Are Depression & Anxiety Connected", 2021). Art is a wonderful way to process your emotions. Of course, if you're just looking for a hobby that is fun, getting creative is for you as well!

Some creative pastimes to consider include:

➢ painting
➢ drawing
➢ dancing
➢ collaging
➢ embroidery
➢ digital art
➢ writing
➢ pottery
➢ baking
➢ gardening
➢ playing a musical instrument

Remember that the end-product doesn't have to be a masterpiece. It doesn't have to be "good enough" for anyone; it just needs to be good for you.

Take Up Journaling

Emotional writing has emotional and physical health benefits (Baikie & Wilhelm, 2005). It is a great way to process your emotions and help you get through difficult situations. Since it helps you express your feelings, it promotes self-awareness, and this can help you discover what you value and what is important to you.

Get Some Fresh Air

Spending time in nature not only decreases stress but also has been scientifically proven to increase feelings of happiness ("Mindful Moment", 2022). I recommend you spend at least two hours outdoors each week. If you don't have time to do it all at once, try breaking it up and spreading it throughout the week, much as you'd do with exercise.

Some fun outdoor activities include:

- hiking
- going to the beach or forest for a picnic
- eating outside
- enjoying a cup of tea in your garden
- heading to the park for a short break
- walking your dog
- walking while listening to a guided meditation

Follow the Sun

Sunlight has many health benefits. Earlier, we learned about circadian rhythm and the role it plays in regulating your sleep. Well, sunlight helps synchronize your circadian rhythm, and as we know, a good night's rest has a positive effect on your mood.

On top of that, sunlight stimulates the release of vitamin D in your body. This vitamin not only helps improve bone density and prevent osteoporosis, but it also combats depression—the enemy of happiness (Anglin et al., 2013).

Listen To Music

Music has the ability to make you happy, especially if it brings back good memories. The right type of music can also relieve stress.

If you're not sure what type of music to listen to, try the following:

➢ If you search for 'happy' or 'upbeat' on music streaming sites, you'll get a playlist of songs that are sure to make you smile.

➢ Listen to some of your favorite songs from a few years back. Nostalgia has a way to lift one's spirits.

➢ What's your favorite movie? Listen to its soundtrack. What you like about the movie might translate to the music too.

➢ Whenever you hear a song that makes you happy, add it to your very own playlist. You can then listen to these songs when you need a mood booster.

Improve Your Relationships

You now have more free time to spend with your loved ones. If you're married or have a long-term partner, you can start paying special attention to them to help them feel cared for and loved. They'll reciprocate, and I can guarantee that this will make you happy.

If you're not in a relationship anymore, there's no time like right now to start looking for love again. Online dating is a great way to meet potential partners. Just beware of scammers who are out to swindle, especially with older women.

One way to feel like a giddy teenager again is to fall in love, and you know what? Love doesn't have an age limit.

Don't forget about your family and friends! Cherish them. If there are any strained relationships, consider sorting things out sooner rather than later. The negative emotions that surround fights with people you care for aren't good for your mental well-being and it has a negative impact on you physically.

See a Therapist

Seeing a therapist can address harmful patterns in your behavior that may be working against your best efforts to embrace life after 50. Therapy can help you become more self-aware, which makes it easier for you to notice self-destructive behavior. In the long run, it contributes to your overall happiness by giving you the tools to manage your mental state and any negative thoughts and feelings.

There's this idea that you need to have at least one mental disorder to see a therapist. That's not the case at all—everyone can benefit from having a chat with a professional.

Practice Gratitude

You'll be surprised how advantageous it is to your overall well-being if you remember the good in your life. It is a brilliant way to get perspective when You're in a rut. By reflecting on the happy moments, the people you appreciate, and what you've achieved in life, you're reminding yourself that good exists even in bad times.

Let's look at some other advantages of being thankful:

> You'll be more satisfied with your life.

> You'll have a more positive disposition.

> You're less likely to suffer from burnout.

> You'll be healthier physically.

> You'll sleep better.

> You'll have more energy.

> The inflammation in your body will decrease.

> You'll be more resilient.

> Your patience will increase.

> You'll be less materialistic.

The above benefits of gratitude were discovered by the Greater Good Science Center in 2018, but another study confirmed their findings and added that gratitude strengthens relationships as well (Emmons & Mishra, 2011).

Gratitude works in four ways (Brown & Wong, 2017):

1. It separates you from negative thoughts, feelings, and self-talk by shifting your attention to positive emotions.

2. It makes us feel more satisfied with life. What's more, you don't have to share your feeling of gratitude with someone for it to benefit you. Merely writing it down can trigger feelings of contentment and happiness.

3. Gratitude compounds like interest. When you start with your gratitude practice, you may not notice the benefits right off the bat. Give it a few weeks and you'll become aware of a shift in your happiness levels and will have a more optimistic outlook.

4. Gratitude trains your brain to be, well, more grateful!

If you're looking to increase your health and happiness, then gratitude is a simple way to do it. Martin Seligman, one of the leaders in the field of positive psychology, believes that "when we take time to notice the things that go right, it means we're getting a lot of little rewards throughout the day" (Brainy Quote, n.d.).

Every time you express gratitude, you get a dopamine boost in your brain that makes you feel good and behave more positively, which makes you feel even better, and so the cycle continues. To keep this sequence going, you have to work at it daily. One of the best ways to practice gratitude is to write it down. To make it a habit, I recommend you create a journal.

Keeping a Gratitude Journal

Considering the benefits of listing what you're grateful for, it makes sense to do it daily to maximize these benefits. Having a journal dedicated to writing down the good things in your life is a smart way to keep all your thoughts in one place. The fact that a journal is easy to carry around with you means you'll have easy access in those moments when you need a reminder that not everything in your life is bad.

The ability to recall even the smallest of moments that brought you joy throughout the day will become second nature the more you force yourself to focus on the good. It takes only a few moments a day, but the advantages of this practice will change the course of your life.

We now have to figure out how to start a gratitude journal you'll actually use. Gratitude journals are similar to the diary you may have kept in your teenage years. The main difference is that you're writing down specifically what you're grateful for and not random thoughts or events about your day.

There's not just one correct way to keep a gratitude journal. The important thing is that you do it daily. I keep my journal next to my computer and have formed a habit of writing in it before I take my shower and prepare for bed. I often fall asleep with a smile on my face. You can imagine how good that is for one's sleep. Other people like writing in their journals first thing in the morning to start their day off on a positive note.

Here are some tips to help get you started on your journey to leading a more appreciative life.

1. Pick a journal

Do you like the feel of a pen in your hand or do you prefer to go digital? Choose the one you know you'll stick to. For example, if you plan on carrying it with you as a reminder during difficult times, then you'll have to choose between paper format and your phone or another portable digital device.

You also have to decide if you're going to use it exclusively as a gratitude journal or a mix of writing down what happened during the day overall. There's also the option of combining your journal with your daily planner. This way, you'll have a constant reminder of all your blessings.

2. Focus on the benefits

Mostly, people don't like doing things without knowing why they're doing them. If you continually remind yourself of the advantages of writing down what You're thankful for, you'll be more likely to do it. A good example is brushing your teeth. You don't always want to do it, but you do it anyway because you know it prevents cavities.

3. Make time

Life sometimes gets ahead of us even in our golden years. I have a few retired friends who seem to be busier now than when they were still working. To make sure that you stick to your daily gratitude journaling, set aside a specific time to do it. Next, set an alarm on your phone as a reminder.

An excellent tip is to always tie a new action you want to turn into a habit to an existing habit. For example, if you enjoy a relaxing cup of coffee in the morning before starting your day, start journaling at the same time. This is a great way to prevent it from feeling like yet another thing to add to your to-do list.

4. Use prompts

It can be hard in the beginning to think of things You're grateful for, especially when you're staring at a blank page. One way to overcome this "gratitude fright" is to use prompts.

Here are a few of my favorite ones:

- ➢ Write about something a loved one did for you.
- ➢ Think about three silly things your children did.
- ➢ Think about the effort that went into making the clothes you're wearing.
- ➢ List three of your most prized possessions.
- ➢ Look outside. Is there something there that you're grateful for?

➤ Go through your photos and pick one randomly. What good things happened at that time?

➤ Write down something you have that you didn't have a year ago.

➤ Write about a time when you laughed so hard you started to cry.

➤ Name three things that made you smile today.

5. Cover Some New Topics

It can be difficult to come up with new things to write about, but as you continue writing in your gratitude journal, you have to get creative, or you'll just repeat the same things over and over again.

One way to keep things fresh is to approach topics from a new angle. For example, if you've already written why you're thankful for your children, try looking at them from an outsider's perspective. You may realize that you're grateful for how positive they are.

It is your gratitude journal, and you're allowed to write about anything. To help you broaden your list of topics, think about the following subjects to help awaken your gratitude muse:

People

- a person who lives far away
- someone you haven't spoken to in a long time.
- your coworkers
- someone you don't like very much
- someone who inspires you
- a kind stranger

Things

- your bedtime routine
- your favorite food
- your job
- your hobbies
- your body
- your senses

Places

- where you like to go on vacation
- your home office
- your bed
- the city you live in
- the park near your home
- your favorite store

Gratitude is a game-changer. Since there is a clear relationship between your mental and physical health, adopting a practice such as gratitude journaling will have an overall positive effect on your well-being. Science backs up the benefits of gratitude.

What I like most about gratitude is that you can put it into practice anywhere. As soon as you find yourself lamenting your age, start thinking about everything you have to be thankful for. Good health, financial stability, a happy marriage, healthy kids, and a silly dog who drools on everything are all good examples. You truly can be grateful for anything—big or small.

At the moment, I am grateful that I'm able to help you overcome whatever ambivalence you may have about life after 50. Knowing that the words I write can positively impact the remainder of your life makes me brim with joy. Thank you for allowing me to walk with you on this journey.

It's not over yet! We still have one chapter to go, and I think you're going to like what you read. It will give you an excuse to go shopping!

Chapter Summary

- ➢ People are living longer, and life expectancy will continue to increase.

- ➢ If you believe your life is over at 50, then it will be.

➤ As you age, your definition of happiness changes; it's less about things and more about authenticity.

➤ Your body and mind influence each other, so you have to take care of your basic needs to be happy.

➤ Don't be afraid of falling in love at 50. Love has no age limit.

➤ Everyone can benefit from having a chat with a therapist.

➤ Expressing gratitude is good for your mind and body.

➤ The more you practice gratitude, the more grateful you'll be.

CHAPTER 8:
THE SECRETS OF ANTI-AGING

Youth are the center of attention in this image-obsessed culture largely bred by social media. Older people, however, are forgotten and often feel lost in a sea of photo-edited perfection.

The first secret of anti-aging? Stop being negative about it! It is absolutely possible to feel younger, healthier, and happier with each passing year.

Innovative research and technology in the field of aging are starting to turn back the hands of time slowly but surely. For example, it was recently discovered that older cells can be 'persuaded' to look and act like their younger equivalents. This form of cell reprogramming can increase a person's lifespan by 30% ("Turning back time", n.d.).

Most Effective Ways to Prevent Aging

While You're waiting for scientists to discover the fountain of youth, there are techniques based on science and smart behavior you can start implementing today to stay looking radiant and glowing.

Dress the Part

If you want to look young, then consider updating your wardrobe. What you wear can take years off your appearance. It's also about being unafraid of wearing the type of clothes you think represent the real you. Embracing your individual style will give you more confidence and you'll go into each day with a spring in your step.

So, how do you dress to look younger but still age appropriately? Admittedly, I have no idea. Thankfully, I'm married to the personification of style. Following my wife's style, I came up with ways that you can use your wardrobe strategically.

Flash Your Wrists

You don't have to make massive changes to dress more youthful yet still be age appropriate. Something as small as rolling up your sleeves can make you look younger. All it takes is a few centimeters of skin to make you look slender, fitter, and more energetic.

This technique works because the wrists are one of the slimmest parts of your body—even if you gain weight your wrists will stay basically the same.

Show Your Ankles

The same principle applies to your ankles (if you're fortunate enough to have skinny ankles). The danger, however, exists that you appear stubbier and shorter if you show too much ankle. You have to make sure that what you're wearing doesn't end on the biggest part of your calf. I suggest you do what my wife does: Parade in front of the mirror. Try a few different styles of pants and see which is more flattering on your body. She often asks my opinion on what she's wearing.

Define Your Waistline

One guaranteed way to rejuvenate your look in an effortless way is to define your waistline. Be careful not to accentuate your waist in an obvious way; it should seem effortless to achieve the desired effect. A good example of effortlessly drawing attention to your waist is tucking in your blouse or shirt.

Accentuate What You Like About Yourself

Everyone has something they like about themselves. If you don't know what that is yet, analyze yourself from head to toe until you find something. For example, if you are particularly fond of your knees, wear skirts to show them off. Similarly, if you think you have a beautiful, long neck, emphasize it by wearing an accessory that compliments it.

Stay On-Trend

To give yourself a youthful, fashion-forward look, add something that is currently trending to your look. Many women feel that if they reach a certain age, they're too old to have an interest in fashion. If you believe that to be true, then I'm glad to be the one who tells you that it isn't. Nothing stops you from following the latest trends and choosing items that inspire you and redress your current wardrobe.

Make Sunscreen Your Best Friend

Unfortunately, the hidden sun damage that occurred 30 years ago will become more visible in your golden years. Hopefully, you applied sunscreen from a young age, but if you didn't, doing so now can slow down possible skin-related conditions, and at best, prevent them from developing at all.

Wear it religiously, even when it is cloudy to protect your skin from harmful UV rays. We will have a more in-depth look at what skincare products you should use to repair your skin a little later on in this chapter.

Start Taking Supplements

With your doctor's approval, start taking supplements and multivitamins that support your body's systems. Vitamin C and

E have many benefits for the skin, bones, and brain. Calcium supports your bone structure and prevents broken bones later in life.

Scientists have identified a number of other substances that promote healthy aging. Here are some of the least known anti-aging substances you can add to your diet.

Curcumin

This may sound like a foreign substance, but you probably already have it in your kitchen—curcumin is the active ingredient in turmeric. Various studies have found that this compound has powerful protective properties right down to the cellular level due to its potent antioxidant abilities (Bielak-Zmijewska et al., 2019).

Curcumin also postpones the onset of age-related ailments and alleviates symptoms if these diseases are already present (Chen et al., 2018).

Turmeric is easy to find, so I recommend you look for ways to add it to the meals you prepare daily. You can also boost your curcumin intake by enjoying an easy-to-make turmeric tea.

You'll need:

- 1 tsp turmeric
- 1 tsp cinnamon
- ½ tsp black pepper
- 1 tbsp honey
- 1 cup water or milk

All that's left to do is bring the water or milk to a boil, add the other ingredients, and let it steep for 10–15 minutes before enjoying this age-defying drink.

If you're not a fan of the taste of turmeric, don't worry. There are various curcumin supplements that come in pill form.

EGCG

Epigallocatechin gallate (EGCG) is known for its impressive health benefits. This polyphenol compound found in green tea reduces your risk of heart disease and certain cancers (Eng et al., 2018). What's even more exciting is that it induces the super anti-aging process we talked about earlier, autophagy (Zang, et al., 2020).

Green tea also comes with its own set of health benefits. Some notable examples include protecting skin against aging and reducing hyperpigmentation caused by UV light (Fukushima et al., 2020).

Collagen

Collagen helps your skin maintain its structure, but as you age, the production of this protein slows down, which leads to lines and wrinkles. One study found that supplementing with 2.5 grams of collagen per day, along with other age-busting ingredients like biotin, improved skin hydration and elasticity (Bolke et al., 2019).

There are various collagen supplements available, including capsules and powders.

CoQ10

Coenzyme Q10 gets released throughout your body naturally. It is a powerful antioxidant that protects against cellular damage. However, as with most things, it declines as you grow older. If you supplement with it, your overall quality of life will improve, you'll have fewer hospital visits, and you'll stay younger physically and mentally.

If you are taking statins to lower high cholesterol, they can cause muscle pain, nausea, liver, and kidney damage, and other complications like increased blood sugar. Statins also lower your body's level of coenzyme Q10, which can cause these side effects to increase.

Nicotinamide Riboside and Nicotinamide Mononucleotide

These two substances are the precursors to nicotinamide adenine dinucleotide (NAD+), which play a crucial role in many bodily functions, including DNA repair, gene expression, and energy metabolism. As you age, levels of this compound decline, opening the door to various age-related diseases. If you restore the NAD+ levels, you can prevent age-associated cellular changes (Mills et al., 2016).

Crocin

The world's most expensive spice, saffron contains crocin, a yellow carotenoid pigment with healing properties. Studies have shown that crocin has superior anti-inflammatory, anti-anxiety, anti-cancer, and antidepressant benefits (Pitsikas, 2015).

Crocin also has a positive impact on skin cells as it reduces inflammation and protects against UV damage.

Considering the high price point of saffron, I recommend you take a concentrated saffron supplement instead.

Dump the Emotional Weight

Emotional baggage can really take a toll on you as you age. Holding on to stress and emotional scars will make you feel years older than you are. Letting go and freeing yourself from the mental weight of any long-term emotional issues is a potent way to change how you feel. And, as we know, your emotional state impacts all areas of your life, so if you want to build healthy habits, dump the weight of trauma, and move on feeling lighter and happier.

Skip Retirement

Many of my friends and colleagues believe retirement to be the final nail in the proverbial coffin. Research tends to agree with them as retirement has been found to cause depression and anxiety, which contributes to premature aging (APA, n.d.).

Retirement isn't for everyone, and some people find it makes them feel directionless and lonely, instead of satisfied and peaceful. The good news is retirement isn't a must. You can continue doing what you love or change course—whatever makes you happy. If you do decide against retirement, just remember to take a vacation every now and again to recharge.

Welcome Change

Older adults are often afraid to make big changes. They feel getting married, moving across the world, studying toward a degree, or switching careers are only meant for the young.

Why limit yourself in such a way? You still have many years left to live, but you have to actually *live* it. You can't sit around and wait to die, too afraid of making life-altering changes. You're the writer of your story; why not make it an adventure?

You now have six more ingredients to add to the ultimate anti-aging recipe. If you find yourself thinking that it's too late to make the necessary changes and implement these age-busting techniques, let me share with you one of my favorite Chinese proverbs: "The best time to plant a tree was 20 years ago. The second-best time is today." Keep this in mind whenever you question your decision to do what you can to get healthy in your 50s.

Thus far, the majority of the anti-aging methods covered in the book are internal. I think it is high time we look at what you can do from the outside. I can't think of a woman who doesn't like to apply lotions and potions to their skin to make it look better. In the next section, we'll look at the anti-aging ingredients you should look for in your skincare products, and more.

Anti-Aging Skincare Routine

First things first: Wrinkles are a natural part of growing older. These folds in your skin are what make you look old. Sadly, when you age, the collagen and elastin in your skin diminish, resulting in thinner skin that is less resistant to damage. When exposed to dehydration, toxins, and other environmental pollutants, wrinkles start to develop and become more pronounced over time.

If you want to slow down the signs of aging, having an effective anti-aging nighttime and daytime skincare routine is a good start.

In general, it is recommended to start using anti-aging products in your 30s. This will give you a head start by maintaining a youthful complexion and slowing down the formation of wrinkles. However, what's one of the mantras of *Aging Gracefully for Women Over 50*? It's never too late to start!

In your 50s, you'll have to focus on using specific ingredients to keep your skin looking young and healthy. Below is a breakdown of the perfect anti-aging skincare routine and the kind of products you should use.

1. Use a cream cleanser.

You should never skip cleansing your face. If you do, the bacteria that inevitably gets onto it throughout the day can lead to clogged pores and a dull and dreary-looking complexion. However, considering that your skin is less elastic and hydrated than it used to be, it is best to use a nourishing cream cleanser, instead of a harsh foaming face wash that will strip your skin of its oils.

When choosing the best cream cleanser, look for one that is gentle yet potent enough to remove all makeup.

2. Don't forget to exfoliate.

Exfoliating your skin is a brilliant way to restore it back to its previous luster. It cleanses, unclogs pores, and boosts circulation. That being said, don't overdo it; you should limit exfoliating to no more than three times a week, less if your skin is extremely thin. Keep a close eye on how your skin responds and modify how many times you exfoliate as well as the products you use until you find something that works for you.

For any skincare routine to classify as anti-aging, it should include exfoliation of some sort. This is because it removes dead skin cells, making way for newer, healthier cells to rise to the top.

Apply a facial serum.

After cleansing your face, it is time to apply a face serum. There are many kinds on the market, so it is up to you to choose one that addresses a specific skin concern you have.

Three of the top age-defying ingredients you want to see in your serum are:

Hyaluronic acid: It helps keep the skin moisturized and hydrated.

Vitamin C: Ascorbic acid is a powerful antioxidant that combats free radicals and helps boost radiance.

Vitamin A/Retinol: It helps improve uneven skin tone, fight pigmentation, and repair texture.

4. Time to moisturize.

When selecting a moisturizer, keep your skin in mind. Do you want to even your skin tone? Or are you looking for something that plumps up wrinkles, making them less obvious? Or do you want to boost your skin's moisture retention for a youthful, dewy, complexion? Whatever you're looking for, there is a product that will suit your needs.

Your moisturizer shouldn't be limited to your face; include your neck and chest area as they're also prone to fine lines.

5. Don't forget your eyes.

To prevent crow's feet and tiny smile lines, you need to use a cream specifically developed for the eyes. Dark circles and under-eye bags can also be treated with the correct eye cream. I remember I had a patient who once told me that she uses a popular hemorrhoid cream under her eyes to remove bags.

Although it may work, I advise against using just anything on such sensitive skin.

6. Start your morning with facial oil.

Natural oil production decreases as you age, so your skin may need a little extra help. By applying a facial oil in the morning, you're locking in moisture, which will make your skin look plumper and hydrated. My wife uses coconut oil all over after her bath or shower to help nourish her skin.

Once You're done applying your skincare, don't forget to use sunscreen to protect your skin from UV damage.

Skincare Ingredients Worth Remembering

The anti-aging industry is a multibillion-dollar industry. With so much money being injected into finding ways to look young, you can rest assured that scientists will continue to push the envelope.

Listed below are some of the top ingredients scientists have pinpointed as anti-aging wonders.

Alpha hydroxy acids (AHAs): The primary purpose of AHAs is to exfoliate the skin. It works by dissolving the dead skin cells, which triggers the skin's natural renewal process. Exfoliating also increases the absorption rate of other products. That is why products containing abrasive ingredients are always used before facial serums and moisturizers.

Beta hydroxy acid (BHA): Much like AHAs, BHA is used to exfoliate the skin. The main difference between the two is that BHA penetrates deeper down. BHA also has antibacterial and anti-inflammatory properties. BHA is labeled as salicylic acid in the ingredient list of skincare products.

Hyaluronic acid: I mentioned hyaluronic acid earlier, but I didn't mention the secret behind this ingredient's popularity. Hyaluronic acid can hold up to 1,000 times its weight in water! When applied to the skin, it attracts water molecules to the surface. This not only hydrates the skin, but it also makes it look smooth. In other words, wrinkles don't appear so deep anymore.

Squalane: This ingredient acts as an emollient, sealing moisture into the skin. It is an offshoot of squalene, a lipid that is naturally present in the skin. Squalane protects the skin from drying out by improving the function of the skin barrier. Not only is that good for the moisture levels of your skin, but it also reduces the severity of wrinkles and prevents the formation of new fine lines.

Polyphenols: This very powerful group of antioxidants can be found in wine, green tea, vegetables, grapes, pomegranate, and many other natural sources. The most common types of polyphenols are tannins, ellagic acid, anthocyanins, and flavonoids. Antioxidants have the important job of fighting off free radicals and protecting the skin from other environmental pollutants that cause wrinkles, fine lines, and sunspots.

Retinol: Probably one of the most popular anti-aging ingredients, retinol (vitamin A), stimulates the production of collagen, increases cell turnover, and improves the skin's ability to heal itself. It improves skin texture by firming it up and promotes an even glow. I do have to mention that many users have experienced redness and flaking after they started using retinol. If this happens to you, check the concentration of the retinol in the product and consider switching to a product that contains a little less. You can move up in intensity as you get used to it. You also have to triple-check to use sunscreen when you use products that contain vitamin A as it can make your skin more sensitive.

Vitamin C: This is, without a doubt, one of the leading skincare ingredients you can find. It is best known for its anti-aging properties, but it can benefit all skin types and skin conditions. Why? Because free radicals and other pollutants don't stand a chance against this potent antioxidant! This ingredient is also appreciated for its skin brightening effect.

Vitamin E: This ingredient is super healing as it repairs skin damage. It is also an antioxidant and will prevent oxidative damage to the skin. Due to its anti-inflammatory effect, vitamin E is often used to soothe irritation. Pairing it with vitamin C creates an antioxidant duo with many anti-aging benefits.

Peptides: Collagen and elastin are proteins in the skin. Peptides are the building blocks of these proteins. If the protein in your skin is happy, then you'll have a healthy-looking complexion. What's more, peptides promote the production of collagen, elastin, and hyaluronic acid. This triggers your skin's natural renewal process. The result? Plumper skin and a reduction in visible lines and wrinkles.

Ferulic acid: This is a popular ingredient in rejuvenating skin care products. It is known to slow down the aging process by preventing oxidative stress and reducing sun damage. When used with vitamins C and E, it improves the stability and efficiency of these antioxidants.

Niacinamide: When it comes to skin brightening, this form of vitamin B3 outshines even vitamin C's abilities. It works by preventing the transfer of pigment and that way, evens out your skin tone. But That's not all this ingredient is known for. It can repair damaged DNA and restore the skin to its previous youthfulness.

The fact that there are so many ingredients proven to prevent, or at the very least, slow down signs of aging is exciting. I can't help but think about the future and all the undiscovered possibilities we're yet to find.

If you take a two-pronged approach to anti-aging—focusing on the inside and outside—the results may surprise you.

In the end, everything works together to create a younger you. Your mindset, what you eat, how you sleep, your clothes, your hair, what you use on your skin; it all affects how you feel about life after 50.

The trick is to maintain the synergy between these various aspects—something that I'm sure you considered impossible to do at first but hopefully now realize is within reach. You just needed the knowledge to understand how aging works and what you could do to put the brakes on it. It's up to you now!

Chapter Summary

> - It's possible to feel younger as you grow older.

> - Innovation in the anti-aging industry makes it more possible with each passing day to turn back the hands of time.

> - Using a mix of behavior and science is the secret to preventing aging.

> - Supplements and vitamins can support your body in its fight against age-related damage.

> - Retirement may not be for you. The good news is that it doesn't have to be.

> - It's not too late to start taking care of your skin.

> - Dehydration, toxins, and environmental pollutants cause your skin to age—but the right ingredients can help!

CONCLUSION

As a 70-year-old, I have had my own fair share of age-related battles. Even as a man, I've stood in front of the mirror not liking what I see. The wrinkles, folds, bags under my eyes, and dull complexion left me feeling out of sorts. Who was this man staring back at me?

Knowing what I know about the ridiculous beauty standards women have to measure up to, I realize that the confusion and frustration I experienced is nowhere near as intense as what they feel.

Aging takes a toll on both genders, but thanks to society and the value we place on external beauty, women have it much harder.

Physical appearance aside, we also must acknowledge the fear and uncertainty that are part of aging. There are suddenly so many age-related diseases we're more at risk of that it's near impossible not to break out in a sweat as we consider the worst.

It was only when I realized how big of an impact my lifestyle choices had on my health and longevity that I started to relax. It was a moment of, "You know what, I'm not completely powerless. I can do X, Y, and Z to give the aging process a run for its money!"

Boy, did I do just that—I beat cancer! I can't think of a better way to show aging who is boss other than overcoming one of the worst things it could throw at me. That is why I decided to write this book. But more than that, I wanted to appeal to female readers specifically. Women are superhuman creatures who still have so many obstacles to overcome—the stigma of reaching midlife being one of them. No, You're not over the hill, frail, pathetic, or worthless.

You're as strong now as you were when you grew a little human in your tummy and gave birth to him or her. You're as strong now as you were when you raised a child, worked a 9–5 job, and somehow managed to cook and clean without losing your mind. Age is just a number, and you shouldn't let society prescribe what you can and can't do when you reach that number.

At its core, *Aging Gracefully for Women Over 50* is about taking back your power. By following the advice written in these pages, you can slow down aging, manage any age-related diseases you may already have, and delay or prevent any other health issues.

Not many women know that following a healthy diet, exercising, sleeping well, and dealing with stress in a mindful manner has such a significant impact on growing older. It's the world's best-kept secret.

In the end, you need to decide what you're willing to do and go for it! I remember when one of my former patients stopped drinking caffeine. That's all. She was 68 at the time and apart from the osteoarthritis, she was fit as a fiddle. Another patient had gone all out. She jumped on the intermittent fasting bandwagon, cut out refined carbs, stopped drinking, and went to the gym four times a week for various classes ranging from dance aerobics to kickboxing to yoga. She was 72 and had been managing her type 2 diabetes with these lifestyle changes.

How extreme you go depends on your lifestyle before 50. If you didn't make the healthiest of choices, you may have to put in a little extra work to get your body to a healthier baseline. If you've been active since a young age, mostly watched what you ate, and didn't stay out partying the whole night too many times, then you may not need to make many changes—you already have healthy habits.

Whatever the case may be, I am confident that you can turn your health around and look and feel better while you do it. Don't underestimate your will to fight for a life worth living. All you need to do is change your mindset from one focused on the negative, to one always searching for the positive.

Let's quickly make a list of all the good things that came from reaching middle age. I'll go first.

> I got cancer and overcame it, and that showed me that I'm stronger than I think.

➢ I was able to live the life I had always dreamed about and see my grandchildren.

➢ I could afford to retire from practice and pursue other hobbies I'm passionate about, like writing this book.

➢ I get to grow old with my best friend and the person I love the most in the world.

I'm interested to see how many positive aspects of life after 50 you listed down. If you find it difficult, keep trying. In time, something good about growing older will enter your mind and I won't be surprised if a smile accompanies it!

Still nothing? Then maybe make a gratitude list first. When You're grateful for what you have, it's much easier to see the positive in any situation.

That, dear reader, brings us to the end of this journey to aging gracefully. I hope this book was of value to you and you learned things that You're excited to apply to your own life. Remember, delaying and even reversing parts of the aging process is as simple as making healthy lifestyle choices. I know you can do it!

But wait, there's more! Read on.

Can you help spread the word?

If you enjoyed this book, and you feel it's helped you in any way, it would mean the world to me if you would please leave a favorable review. I'm on a quest to get 500 reviews and could really use your help so I could impact more lives. Also, share it with your friends if you think they may benefit from it. The sooner we can change the stigma attached to aging, the easier it will be for future generations to age gracefully.

Click the link below to post your review on Amazon.

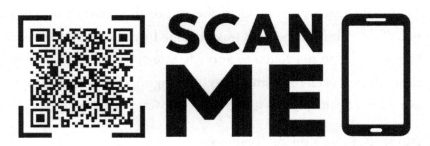

https://www.amazon.com/review/create-review/error?&asinB0B6XX3CVC

BOOK DESCRIPTION OF
MY UPCOMING BOOK:

INTERMITTENT FASTING
FOR WOMEN OVER 50:

Dr. Steve's Guide for Rapid Weight Loss, Energy, Detoxification, Diabetes and Anti-Aging

Are you tired of being tired? Has life over 50 taken the wind out of your sails by adding a few extra pounds? Do thoughts of your ailing health keep you up at night? If so, then Dr. Steve's ultimate guide for rapid weight loss, energy, detoxification, and anti-aging is here to help.

Dr. Steve knows you don't want to crash diet, but instead want to improve your overall health by making key lifestyle changes. To help you do just that, he wrote *Intermittent Fasting for Women Over 50*. This book will show you how time-restricted eating can help you lose weight, feel more energized, and improve your general health. There are no gimmicks, fads, or 'miracle' pills involved. Intermittent fasting is a simple way to shrink down your waist, improve your health markers, and add years to your life without you having to experience any discomfort.

The fact is that your body needs a little help when you get older. Menopause causes a lot of changes in a woman's body and with that comes many side effects. The good news is that IF has been scientifically proven to help get women through menopause and out the other side smiling.

In *Intermittent Fasting for Women Over 50*, you will learn:

> - Why IF is considered the closest thing to the fountain of youth we currently have.
> - How IF works, complete with scientific proof to back up all the health claims.
> - The different types of IF protocols there are and how to choose one to fit in with your life.
> - How your mindset plays a vital role in how you approach life after 50.
> - What foods you should avoid if you want to improve your health and lose weight.
> - How even moderate exercise can have life-changing effects on your overall well-being.
> - How you can pair IF with the ketogenic diet, veganism, or any other eating plan you may already be on.
> - And much, much more.

Dr. Steve is in his 70s, retired, and a cancer survivor. He is passionate about reversing the aging process and reducing disease using a combination of diet, fitness, and naturally boosting the immune system. His previous book, *Aging Gracefully for Women Over 50* has been lauded as a must-read for women over 50 who don't want to give up on life because they're 'old.' In fact, Dr. Steve has through the course of his career and through his first book helped many women accept that life begins at 50; it's just up to them to make the right choices!

After reading *Intermittent Fasting for Women Over 50*, he hopes your vigor for life will be restored and you'll go on to live a healthy and happy life.

REFERENCES

Ahmed, A., Saeed, F., Arshad, M. U., Afzaal, M., Imran, A., Ali, S. W., Niaz, B., Ahmad, A., & Imran, M. (2018). Impact of intermittent fasting on human health: an extended review of metabolic cascades. International Journal of Food Properties, 21(1), 2700–2713. https://doi.org/10.1080/10942912.2018.1560312

Alesio, G. (2018, September 17). Roles of Insulin in the Human Body. Profolus. https://www.profolus.com/topics/roles-of-insulin-in-the-human-body/

Altman, B. J., & Rathmell, J. C. (2009). Autophagy: Not good OR bad, but good AND bad. Autophagy, 5(4), 569–570. https://doi.org/10.4161/auto.5.4.8254

Altman, D. (2019, August 7). The Single Word That Stops Negative Self-Talk | Psychology Today. www.psychologytoday.com. https://www.psychologytoday.com/us/blog/practical-mindfulness/201908/the-single-word-stops-negative-self-talk

Amaravadi, R. K., Kimmelman, A. C., & Debnath, J. (2019). Targeting Autophagy in Cancer: Recent Advances and Future Directions. Cancer Discovery, 9(9), 1167–1181. https://doi.org/10.1158/2159-8290.cd-19-0292

Anglin, R. E. S., Samaan, Z., Walter, S. D., & McDonald, S. D. (2013). Vitamin D deficiency and depression in adults: systematic review and meta-analysis. British Journal of Psychiatry, 202(2), 100–107. https://doi.org/10.1192/bjp.bp.111.106666

Annamarya Scaccia. (2018, May 16). How Long Do Symptoms of Menopause Last? Healthline; Healthline Media. https://www.healthline.com/health/menopause/how-long-does-menopause-last

Anothaisintawee, T., Reutrakul, S., Van Cauter, E., & Thakkinstian, A. (2016). Sleep disturbances compared to traditional risk factors for diabetes development: Systematic review and meta-analysis. Sleep Medicine Reviews, 30, 11–24. https://doi.org/10.1016/j.smrv.2015.10.002

Are Depression and Creativity Connected? (2021, November 2). Psych Central. https://psychcentral.com/depression/creativity-and-depression

Arrieta, H., Rezola-Pardo, C., Gil, S. M., Virgala, J., Iturburu, M., Antón, I., González-Templado, V., Irazusta, J., & Rodriguez-Larrad, A. (2019). Effects of Multicomponent Exercise on Frailty in Long-Term Nursing Homes: A Randomized Controlled Trial. Journal of the American Geriatrics Society, 67(6), 1145–1151. https://doi.org/10.1111/jgs.15824

Arsenis, N. C., You, T., Ogawa, E. F., Tinsley, G. M., & Zuo, L. (2017). Physical activity and telomere length: Impact of aging and potential mechanisms of action. Oncotarget, 8(27). https://doi.org/10.18632/oncotarget.16726

APA. (n.d.). Retiring minds want to know. https://www.apa.org/monitor/2014/01/retiring-minds

Bacaro, V., Ballesio, A., Cerolini, S., Vacca, M., Poggiogalle, E., Donini, L. M., Lucidi, F., & Lombardo, C. (2020). Sleep duration and obesity in adulthood: An updated systematic review and meta-analysis. Obesity Research & Clinical Practice, 14(4), 301–309. https://doi.org/10.1016/j.orcp.2020.03.004

Bagherniya, M., Butler, A. E., Barreto, G. E., & Sahebkar, A. (2018). The effect of fasting or calorie restriction on autophagy induction: A review of the literature. Ageing Research Reviews, 47, 183–197. https://doi.org/10.1016/j.arr.2018.08.004

Baik, S.-H., Rajeev, V., Fann, D. Y.-W., Jo, D.-G., & Arumugam, T. V. (2020). Intermittent fasting increases adult hippocampal neurogenesis. Brain and Behavior, 10(1), e01444. https://doi.org/10.1002/brb3.1444

Baikie, K. A., & Wilhelm, K. (2005). Emotional and physical health benefits of expressive writing. Advances in Psychiatric Treatment, 11(5), 338–346. https://doi.org/10.1192/apt.11.5.338

Barnosky, A. R., Hoddy, K. K., Unterman, T. G., & Varady, K. A. (2014). Intermittent fasting vs daily calorie restriction for type 2 diabetes prevention: a review of human findings. Translational Research, 164(4), 302–311. https://doi.org/10.1016/j.trsl.2014.05.013

Battaglia Richi, E., Baumer, B., Conrad, B., Darioli, R., Schmid, A., & Keller, U. (2015). Health Risks Associated with Meat Consumption: A Review of Epidemiological Studies. International Journal for Vitamin and Nutrition Research. Internationale Zeitschrift Fur Vitamin- Und Ernahrungsforschung. Journal International de Vitaminologie et de Nutrition, 85(1-2), 70–78. https://doi.org/10.1024/0300-9831/a000224

Bielak-Zmijewska, A., Grabowska, W., Ciolko, A., Bojko, A., Mosieniak, G., Bijoch, Ł., & Sikora, E. (2019). The Role of Curcumin in the Modulation of Ageing. International Journal of Molecular Sciences, 20(5), 1239. https://doi.org/10.3390/ijms20051239

Bilsborough, S. A., & Crowe, T. C. (2003). Low-carbohydrate diets: what are the potential short- and long-term health implications? Asia Pacific Journal of Clinical Nutrition, 12(4), 396–404. https://pubmed.ncbi.nlm.nih.gov/14672862/

Bolke, L., Schlippe, G., Gerß, J., & Voss, W. (2019). A Collagen Supplement Improves Skin Hydration, Elasticity, Roughness, and Density: Results of a Randomized, Placebo-Controlled, Blind Study. Nutrients, 11(10), 2494. https://doi.org/10.3390/nu11102494

Bondonno, N. P., Dalgaard, F., Kyrø, C., Murray, K., Bondonno, C. P., Lewis, J. R., Croft, K. D., Gislason, G., Scalbert, A., Cassidy, A., Tjønneland, A., Overvad, K., & Hodgson, J. M. (2019). Flavonoid intake is associated with lower mortality in the Danish Diet Cancer and Health Cohort. Nature Communications, 10(1), 3651. https://doi.org/10.1038/s41467-019-11622-x

Bone Health and Osteoporosis. Osteoporosis Fast Facts. (2015). http://www.bonehealthandosteoporosis.org/wp-content/uploads/2015/12/Osteoporosis-Fast-Facts.pdf

Brown, J., & Wong, J. (2017, June 6). How Gratitude Changes You and Your Brain. Greater Good. https://greatergood.berkeley.edu/article/item/how_gratit ude_changes_you_and_your_brain

Brum, M. C. B., Dantas Filho, F. F., Schnorr, C. C., Bertoletti, O. A., Bottega, G. B., & da Costa Rodrigues, T. (2020). Night shift work, short sleep and obesity. Diabetology & Metabolic Syndrome, 12(1). https://doi.org/10.1186/s13098-020-0524-9

CDC. (2017). CDC - Data and Statistics - Sleep and Sleep Disorders. Centers for Disease Control and Prevention. https://www.cdc.gov/sleep/data_statistics.html

CDC. (2019). National Diabetes Statistics Report. Center for Disease Control and Prevention. https://www.cdc.gov/diabetes/data/statistics-report/index.html

Chen, Y., Liu, X., Jiang, C., Liu, L., Ordovas, J. M., Lai, C., & Shen, L. (2018). Curcumin supplementation increases survival and lifespan in Drosophila under heat stress conditions. BioFactors, 44(6), 577–587. https://doi.org/10.1002/biof.1454

Chiba, Y., Saitoh, S., Takagi, S., Ohnishi, H., Katoh, N., Ohata, J., Nakagawa, M., & Shimamoto, K. (2007). Relationship between Visceral Fat and Cardiovascular Disease Risk Factors: The Tanno and Sobetsu Study. Hypertension Research, 30(3), 229–236. https://doi.org/10.1291/hypres.30.229

Conklin, Q. A., King, B. G., Zanesco, A. P., Lin, J., Hamidi, A. B., Pokorny, J. J., Álvarez-López, M. J., Cosín-Tomás, M., Huang, C., Kaliman, P., Epel, E. S., & Saron, C. D. (2018). Insight meditation and telomere biology: The effects of intensive retreat and the moderating role of personality. Brain, Behavior, and Immunity, 70, 233–245. https://doi.org/10.1016/j.bbi.2018.03.003

Conway, S.-M. (2020, January 8). How Does Intermittent Fasting Affect Our Brain Health? Simple.life Blog. https://simple.life/blog/intermittent-fasting-for-brain-health/

de Cabo, R., & Mattson, M. P. (2019). Effects of Intermittent Fasting on Health, Aging, and Disease. New England Journal of Medicine, 381(26), 2541–2551. https://doi.org/10.1056/nejmra1905136

Ding, C., Lim, L. L., Xu, L., & Kong, A. P. S. (2018). Sleep and Obesity. Journal of Obesity & Metabolic Syndrome, 27(1), 4–24. https://doi.org/10.7570/jomes.2018.27.1.4

Dionigi, R. A. (2015). Stereotypes of Aging: Their Effects on the Health of Older Adults. Journal of Geriatrics, 2015, 1–9. https://doi.org/10.1155/2015/954027

Dong, T. A., Sandesara, P. B., Dhindsa, D. S., Mehta, A., Arneson, L. C., Dollar, A. L., Taub, P. R., & Sperling, L. S. (2020). Intermittent Fasting: A Heart Healthy Dietary Pattern? The American Journal of Medicine, 133(8). https://doi.org/10.1016/j.amjmed.2020.03.030

Dreher, M. L., & Davenport, A. J. (2013). Hass Avocado Composition and Potential Health Effects. Critical Reviews in Food Science and Nutrition, 53(7), 738–750. https://doi.org/10.1080/10408398.2011.556759

Emmons, R. A., & Mishra, A. (2011). Why gratitude enhances well-being: What we know, what we need to know. In K. M. Sheldon, T. B. Kashdan, & M. F. Steger (Eds.), Series in positive psychology. Designing positive psychology: Taking stock and moving forward(pp. 248-262). New York, NY, US: Oxford University Press. https://emmons.faculty.ucdavis.edu/wp–content/uploads/sites/90/2015/08/2011_2-16_Sheldon_Chapter-16-11.pdf

Eng, Q. Y., Thanikachalam, P. V., & Ramamurthy, S. (2018). Molecular understanding of Epigallocatechin gallate (EGCG) in cardiovascular and metabolic diseases. Journal of Ethnopharmacology, 210, 296–310. https://doi.org/10.1016/j.jep.2017.08.035

Epel, E. S., Blackburn, E. H., Lin, J., Dhabhar, F. S., Adler, N. E., Morrow, J. D., & Cawthon, R. M. (2004). Accelerated telomere shortening in response to life stress. Proceedings of the National Academy of Sciences, 101(49), 17312–17315. https://doi.org/10.1073/pnas.0407162101

Epel, E., Daubenmier, J., Moskowitz, J. T., Folkman, S., & Blackburn, E. (2009). Can Meditation Slow Rate of Cellular Aging? Cognitive Stress, Mindfulness, and Telomeres. Annals of the New York Academy of Sciences, 1172(1), 34–53. https://doi.org/10.1111/j.1749-6632.2009.04414.x

Erickson, K. I., Hillman, C., Stillman, C. M., Ballard, R. M., Bloodgood, B., Conroy, D. E., Macko, R., Marquez, D. X., Petruzzello, S. J., & Powell, K. E. (2019). Physical Activity, Cognition, and Brain Outcomes. Medicine & Science in Sports & Exercise, 51(6), 1242–1251. https://doi.org/10.1249/mss.0000000000001936

Expanding the Science and Practice of Gratitude. (2018). Ggsc.berkeley.edu. https://ggsc.berkeley.edu/what_we_do/major_initiatives/expanding_gratitude

FastStats - Osteoporosis. (2019). Centers for Disease Control and Prevention. https://www.cdc.gov/nchs/fastats/osteoporosis.htm

Fiedor, J., & Burda, K. (2014). Potential Role of Carotenoids as Antioxidants in Human Health and Disease. Nutrients, 6(2), 466–488. https://doi.org/10.3390/nu6020466

Foley, D. J., Monjan, A. A., Brown, S. L., Simonsick, E. M., Wallace, R. B., & Blazer, D. G. (1995). Sleep Complaints Among Elderly Persons: An Epidemiologic Study of Three Communities. Sleep, 18(6), 425–432. https://doi.org/10.1093/sleep/18.6.425

Fukushima, Y., Takahashi, Y., Kishimoto, Y., Taguchi, C., Suzuki, N., Yokoyama, M., & Kondo, K. (2020). Consumption of Polyphenols in Coffee and Green Tea Alleviates Skin Photoaging in Healthy Japanese Women. Clinical, Cosmetic and Investigational Dermatology, Volume 13, 165–172. https://doi.org/10.2147/ccid.s225043

Fung, J. (2016, October 5). How to renew your body: Fasting and autophagy. Diet Doctor. https://www.dietdoctor.com/renew-body-fasting-autophagy

Gagne, D. A., Von Holle, A., Brownley, K. A., Runfola, C. D., Hofmeier, S., Branch, K. E., & Bulik, C. M. (2012). Eating disorder symptoms and weight and shape concerns in a large web-based convenience sample of women ages 50 and above: results of the Gender and Body Image (GABI) study. The International Journal of Eating Disorders, 45(7), 832–844. https://doi.org/10.1002/eat.22030

Gaines, J. (2020, November 17). The Philosophy of Ikigai: 3 Examples About Finding Purpose. PositivePsychology.com. https://positivepsychology.com/ikigai/

Gill, C. I., Haldar, S., Boyd, L. A., Bennett, R., Whiteford, J., Butler, M., Pearson, J. R., Bradbury, I., & Rowland, I. R. (2007). Watercress supplementation in diet reduces lymphocyte DNA damage and alters blood antioxidant status in healthy adults. The American Journal of Clinical Nutrition, 85(2), 504–510. https://doi.org/10.1093/ajcn/85.2.504

Glick, D., Barth, S., & Macleod, K. F. (2010). Autophagy: cellular and molecular mechanisms. The Journal of Pathology, 221(1), 3–12. https://doi.org/10.1002/path.2697

Goodrick, C. L., Ingram, D. K., Reynolds, M. A., Freeman, J. R., & Cider, N. L. (1982). Effects of intermittent feeding upon growth and life span in rats. Gerontology, 28(4), 233–241. https://doi.org/10.1159/000212538

Gooley, J. J., Chamberlain, K., Smith, K. A., Khalsa, S. B. S., Rajaratnam, S. M. W., Van Reen, E., Zeitzer, J. M., Czeisler, C. A., & Lockley, S. W. (2011). Exposure to Room Light before Bedtime Suppresses Melatonin Onset and Shortens Melatonin Duration in Humans. The Journal of Clinical Endocrinology & Metabolism, 96(3), E463–E472. https://doi.org/10.1210/jc.2010-2098

Gottberg, K. (2015, September 28). What Carl Jung Teaches Us About The Art Of Aging Well. HuffPost. https://www.huffpost.com/entry/carl-jung-aging_b_8173372

Gotter, A. (2018, April 20). What Is the 4-7-8 Breathing Technique? Healthline; Healthline Media. https://www.healthline.com/health/4-7-8-breathing

Guerrero, F. A., & Medina, G. M. (2017). Effect of a medicinal plant (Passiflora incarnata L) on sleep. Sleep Science, 10(3), 96–100. https://doi.org/10.5935/1984-0063.20170018

Guo, E. L., & Katta, R. (2017). Diet and hair loss: effects of nutrient deficiency and supplement use. Dermatology Practical & Conceptual, 7(1), 1–10. https://doi.org/10.5826/dpc.0701a01

Havighurst, R. J. (1961). Successful aging. The Gerontologist, 1(1), 8–13. https://doi.org/10.1093/geront/1.1.8

Hays, J. C., Blazer, D. G., & Foley, D. J. (1996). Risk of Napping: Excessive Daytime Sleepiness and Mortality in an Older Community Population. Journal of the American Geriatrics Society, 44(6), 693–698. https://doi.org/10.1111/j.1532-5415.1996.tb01834.x

Ho, H. V. T., Jovanovski, E., Zurbau, A., Blanco Mejia, S., Sievenpiper, J. L., Au-Yeung, F., Jenkins, A. L., Duvnjak, L., Leiter, L., & Vuksan, V. (2017). A systematic review and meta-analysis of randomized controlled trials of the effect of konjac glucomannan, a viscous soluble fiber, on LDL cholesterol and the new lipid targets non-HDL cholesterol and apolipoprotein B. The American Journal of Clinical Nutrition, 105(5), 1239–1247. https://doi.org/10.3945/ajcn.116.142158

Horne, B. D., Muhlestein, J. B., & Anderson, J. L. (2015). Health effects of intermittent fasting: hormesis or harm? A systematic review. The American Journal of Clinical Nutrition, 102(2), 464–470. https://doi.org/10.3945/ajcn.115.109553

https://www.facebook.com/BlueZones. (2015). History of Blue Zones - Blue Zones. Blue Zones. https://www.bluezones.com/about/history/

Irwin, M. R. (2019). Sleep and inflammation: partners in sickness and in health. Nature Reviews Immunology, 19(11). https://doi.org/10.1038/s41577-019-0190-z

Johansson, P., Dahlström, Ö., Dahlström, U., & Alehagen, U. (2015). Improved health-related quality of life, and more days out of hospital with supplementation with selenium and coenzyme Q10 combined. Results from a double blind, placebo-controlled prospective study. The Journal of Nutrition, Health & Aging, 19(9), 870–877. https://doi.org/10.1007/s12603-015-0509-9

Jordan, S., Tung, N., Casanova-Acebes, M., Chang, C., Cantoni, C., Zhang, D., Wirtz, T. H., Naik, S., Rose, S. A., Brocker, C. N., Gainullina, A., Hornburg, D., Horng, S., Maier, B. B., Cravedi, P., LeRoith, D., Gonzalez, F. J., Meissner, F., Ochando, J., & Rahman, A. (2019). Dietary Intake Regulates the Circulating Inflammatory Monocyte Pool. Cell, 178(5), 1102-1114.e17. https://doi.org/10.1016/j.cell.2019.07.050

Kalyani, R. R., Corriere, M., & Ferrucci, L. (2014). Age-related and disease-related muscle loss: the effect of diabetes, obesity, and other diseases. The Lancet. Diabetes & Endocrinology, 2(10), 819–829. https://doi.org/10.1016/S2213-8587(14)70034-8

Kernisan, L. (2015, October 1). 4 Brain-Slowing Medications to Avoid if You're Worried About Memory. Better Health While Aging. https://betterhealthwhileaging.net/medications-to-avoid-if-worried-about-memory/

Kinderman, P., Schwannauer, M., Pontin, E., & Tai, S. (2013). Psychological Processes Mediate the Impact of Familial Risk, Social Circumstances and Life Events on Mental Health. PLoS ONE, 8(10), e76564. https://doi.org/10.1371/journal.pone.0076564

Krittanawong, C., Tunhasiriwet, A., Wang, Z., Zhang, H., Farrell, A. M., Chirapongsathorn, S., Sun, T., Kitai, T., & Argulian, E. (2017). Association between short and long sleep durations and cardiovascular outcomes: a systematic review and meta-analysis. European Heart Journal: Acute Cardiovascular Care, 8(8), 762–770. https://doi.org/10.1177/2048872617741733

Lai, H.-L. ., Chang, E.-T. ., Li, Y.-M. ., Huang, C.-Y. ., Lee, L.-H. ., & Wang, H.-M. . (2014). Effects of Music Videos on Sleep Quality in Middle-Aged and Older Adults With Chronic Insomnia: A Randomized Controlled Trial. Biological Research for Nursing, 17(3), 340–347. https://doi.org/10.1177/1099800414549237

Lavin, K. M., Roberts, B. M., S. Fry., Moro, T., Rasmussen, B. B., & Bamman, M. M. (2019). The importance of resistance exercise training to combat neuromuscular aging. The International Union of Physiological Sciences, https://journals.physiology.org/doi/epdfplus/10.1152/physiol.00044.2018

Legg, T.J. (2018). What is the 4-7-8 breathing technique? Healthline. https://www.healthline.com/health/4-7-8-breathing

Lindseth, G., & Murray, A. (2016). Dietary Macronutrients and Sleep. Western Journal of Nursing Research, 38(8), 938–958. https://doi.org/10.1177/0193945916643712

Lowering Cholesterol with a Plant-Based Diet. (2000). Physicians Committee for Responsible Medicine. https://www.pcrm.org/good-nutrition/nutrition-information/lowering-cholesterol-with-a-plant-based-diet

Luglio, H. F. (2014). Estrogen and body weight regulation in women: the role of estrogen receptor alpha (ER-α) on adipocyte lipolysis. Acta Med Indones, 46(4), 333–8. https://pubmed.ncbi.nlm.nih.gov/25633552/

Makarem, N., Shechter, A., Carnethon, M. R., Mullington, J. M., Hall, M. H., & Abdalla, M. (2019). Sleep Duration and Blood Pressure: Recent Advances and Future Directions. Current Hypertension Reports, 21(5). https://doi.org/10.1007/s11906-019-0938-7

Martin Seligman Quotes. (n.d.). BrainyQuote. Retrieved May 17, 2022, from https://www.brainyquote.com/authors/martin_seligman

Martin, P., Kelly, N., Kahana, B., Kahana, E., Willcox, B. J., Willcox, D. C., & Poon, L. W. (2014). Defining Successful Aging: A Tangible or Elusive Concept? The Gerontologist, 55(1), 14–25. https://doi.org/10.1093/geront/gnu044

Mattson, M. P., Moehl, K., Ghena, N., Schmaedick, M., & Cheng, A. (2018). Intermittent metabolic switching, neuroplasticity and brain health. Nature Reviews Neuroscience, 19(2), 80–80. https://doi.org/10.1038/nrn.2017.156

McCarty, R. (2016, December 31). The Fight-or-Flight Response. ResearchGate; unknown. https://www.researchgate.net/publication/303791689_The_Fight-or-Flight_Response

McMahon, D. (2017). A Brief History of Happiness [YouTube Video]. In YouTube. https://www.youtube.com/watch?v=zTnFbWzJzIM

Messina, M. (2016). Impact of Soy Foods on the Development of Breast Cancer and the Prognosis of Breast Cancer Patients. Complementary Medicine Research, 23(2), 75–80. https://doi.org/10.1159/000444735

Mills, K. F., Yoshida, S., Stein, L. R., Grozio, A., Kubota, S., Sasaki, Y., Redpath, P., Migaud, M. E., Apte, R. S., Uchida, K., Yoshino, J., & Imai, S. (2016). Long-Term Administration of Nicotinamide Mononucleotide Mitigates Age-Associated Physiological Decline in Mice. Cell Metabolism, 24(6), 795–806. https://doi.org/10.1016/j.cmet.2016.09.013

Mindful Moment: How Nature Can Heal the Mind and Body. (2022, April 7). Psych Central. https://psychcentral.com/health/mindful-moment-how-nature-can-heal-the-body-and-mind

Mitchell, S. J., Bernier, M., Mattison, J. A., Aon, M. A., Kaiser, T. A., Anson, R. M., Ikeno, Y., Anderson, R. M., Ingram, D. K., & de Cabo, R. (2019). Daily Fasting Improves Health and Survival in Male Mice Independent of Diet Composition and Calories. Cell Metabolism, 29(1), 221-228.e3. https://doi.org/10.1016/j.cmet.2018.08.011

Mohamed, S.K. (2012). Antioxidant and immunostimulant effect of carica papaya linn. Aqueous extract in acrylamide intoxicated rats. *Journal of the Society for Medical Informatics of Bosnia & Herzegovina, 20*(3), 180–185. https://doi.org/10.5455/aim.2012.20.180–185

National Osteoporosis Foundation. (2015). *Osteoporosis fast facts.* http://www.bonehealthandosteoporosis.org/wp-content/uploads/2015/12/Osteoporosis-Fast-Facts.pdf

Nettleton, J. A., Brouwer, I. A., Mensink, R. P., Diekman, C., & Hornstra, G. (2018). Fats in Foods: Current Evidence for Dietary Advice. Annals of Nutrition & Metabolism, 72(3), 248–254. https://doi.org/10.1159/000488006

Neugarten, B. (1996). The Meanings of Age. In press.uchicago.edu. The University of Chicago Press. https://press.uchicago.edu/ucp/books/book/chicago/M/bo3616629.html#anchor-excerpt

Oeppen, J. (2002). DEMOGRAPHY: Enhanced: Broken Limits to Life Expectancy. Science, 296(5570), 1029–1031. https://doi.org/10.1126/science.1069675

Okano, K., Kaczmarzyk, J. R., Dave, N., Gabrieli, J. D. E., & Grossman, J. C. (2019). Sleep quality, duration, and consistency are associated with better academic performance in college students. Npj Science of Learning, 4(1). https://doi.org/10.1038/s41539-019-0055-z

Older Adults' Health. (2021). Apa.org. https://www.apa.org/advocacy/health/older-americans

Orenstein, G. A., & Lewis, L. (2021, November 14). Eriksons stages of psychosocial development. PubMed; StatPearls Publishing. https://www.ncbi.nlm.nih.gov/books/NBK556096/

Park, S. Y., Oh, M. K., Lee, B. S., Kim, H. G., Lee, W. J., Lee, J. H., Lim, J. T., & Kim, J. Y. (2015). The Effects of Alcohol on Quality of Sleep. Korean journal of family medicine, 36(6), 294–299. https://doi.org/10.4082/kjfm.2015.36.6.294

Partial sleep deprivation linked to biological aging in older adults. (2015, June 10). American Academy of Sleep Medicine – Association for Sleep Clinicians and Researchers. https://aasm.org/partial-sleep-deprivation-linked-to-biological-aging-in-older-adults/

Patterson, R. E., & Sears, D. D. (2017). Metabolic Effects of Intermittent Fasting. Annual Review of Nutrition, 37(1), 371–393. https://doi.org/10.1146/annurev-nutr-071816-064634

Pitsikas, N. (2015). The Effect ofCrocus sativusL. and Its Constituents on Memory: Basic Studies and Clinical Applications. Evidence-Based Complementary and Alternative Medicine, 2015, 1–7. https://doi.org/10.1155/2015/926284

Pizzino, G., Irrera, N., Cucinotta, M., Pallio, G., Mannino, F., Arcoraci, V., Squadrito, F., Altavilla, D., & Bitto, A. (2017). Oxidative Stress: Harms and Benefits for Human Health. Oxidative Medicine and Cellular Longevity, 2017(8416763), 1–13. https://doi.org/10.1155/2017/8416763

Ponte Márquez, P. H., Feliu-Soler, A., Solé-Villa, M. J., Matas-Pericas, L., Filella-Agullo, D., Ruiz-Herrerias, M., Soler-Ribaudi, J., Roca-Cusachs Coll, A., & Arroyo-Díaz, J. A. (2018). Benefits of mindfulness meditation in reducing blood pressure and stress in patients with arterial hypertension. Journal of Human Hypertension, 33(3), 237–247. https://doi.org/10.1038/s41371-018-0130-6

Pregnancy Calendar: Your Pregnancy Week-by-Week | What to Expect. (2018, January 10). Whattoexpect. https://www.whattoexpect.com/pregnancy/week-by-week/

Publishing, H. H. (2013, July 1). Add color to your diet for good nutrition. Harvard Health. https://www.health.harvard.edu/staying-healthy/add-color-to-your-diet-for-good-nutrition

Retiring minds want to know. (n.d.). Https://Www.apa.org. https://www.apa.org/monitor/2014/01/retiring-minds

Robertson, D. A., King-Kallimanis, B. L., & Kenny, R. A. (2016). Negative perceptions of aging predict longitudinal decline in cognitive function. Psychology and Aging, 31(1), 71–81. https://doi.org/10.1037/pag0000061

Romeijn, N., Raymann, R. J. E. M., Møst, E., Te Lindert, B., Van Der Meijden, W. P., Fronczek, R., Gomez-Herrero, G., & Van Someren, E. J. W. (2011). Sleep, vigilance, and thermosensitivity. Pflügers Archiv - European Journal of Physiology, 463(1), 169–176. https://doi.org/10.1007/s00424-011-1042-2

Ros, E. (2010). Health Benefits of Nut Consumption. Nutrients, 2(7), 652–682. https://doi.org/10.3390/nu2070652

Ruegsegger, G. N., & Booth, F. W. (2018). Health Benefits of Exercise. Cold Spring Harbor Perspectives in Medicine, 8(7), a029694. https://doi.org/10.1101/cshperspect.a029694

Sadek, K. (2012). Antioxidant and Immunostimulant Effect of Carica Papaya Linn. Aqueous Extract in Acrylamide Intoxicated Rats. Acta Informatica Medica, 20(3), 180. https://doi.org/10.5455/aim.2012.20.180-185

Schagen, S. K., Zampeli, V. A., Makrantonaki, E., & Zouboulis, C. C. (2012). Discovering the link between nutrition and skin aging. Dermato-Endocrinology, 4(3), 298–307. https://doi.org/10.4161/derm.22876

Shea, M. K., Booth, S. L., Massaro, J. M., Jacques, P. F., D'Agostino, R. B., Sr, Dawson-Hughes, B., Ordovas, J. M., O'Donnell, C. J., Kathiresan, S., Keaney, J. F., Jr, Vasan, R. S., & Benjamin, E. J. (2008). Vitamin K and Vitamin D Status: Associations with Inflammatory Markers in the Framingham Offspring Study. American Journal of Epidemiology, 167(3), 313–320. https://doi.org/10.1093/aje/kwm306

Skrovankova, S., Sumczynski, D., Mlcek, J., Jurikova, T., & Sochor, J. (2015). Bioactive Compounds and Antioxidant Activity in Different Types of Berries. International Journal of Molecular Sciences, 16(10), 24673–24706. https://doi.org/10.3390/ijms161024673

St-Onge, M.-P., Mikic, A., & Pietrolungo, C. E. (2016). Effects of Diet on Sleep Quality. Advances in Nutrition, 7(5), 938–949. https://doi.org/10.3945/an.116.012336

Stahl, W., & Sies, H. (2012). β-Carotene and other carotenoids in protection from sunlight. The American Journal of Clinical Nutrition, 96(5), 1179S84S. https://doi.org/10.3945/ajcn.112.034819

The Irish Longitudinal Study on Ageing (TILDA) - Trinity College Dublin. (2016). Tilda.tcd.ie. https://tilda.tcd.ie/news-events/2016/1603-ageing-perceptions-attitudes/

Tobacco and Cancer | CDC. (2021, November 18).
Www.cdc.gov.
https://www.cdc.gov/cancer/tobacco/index.htm#:~:text=
Smokeless%20tobacco%20products%2C%20such%20as
%20dipping%20and%20chewing

Trockel, M. T., Menon, N. K., Rowe, S. G., Stewart, M. T.,
Smith, R., Lu, M., Kim, P. K., Quinn, M. A., Lawrence,
E., Marchalik, D., Farley, H., Normand, P., Felder, M.,
Dudley, J. C., & Shanafelt, T. D. (2020). Assessment of
Physician Sleep and Wellness, Burnout, and Clinically
Significant Medical Errors. JAMA Network Open, 3(12),
e2028111.
https://doi.org/10.1001/jamanetworkopen.2020.28111

Turning back time: Salk scientists reverse signs of aging. (n.d.).
Salk Institute for Biological Studies.
https://www.salk.edu/news-release/turning-back-time-
salk-scientists-reverse-signs-aging/

Tyagi, S., Resnick, N. M., Perera, S., Monk, T. H., Hall, M. H., &
Buysse, D. J. (2014). Behavioral Treatment of Insomnia:
Also Effective for Nocturia. Journal of the American
Geriatrics Society, 62(1), 54–60.
https://doi.org/10.1111/jgs.12609

USDA. (2020). Dietary Guidelines for Americans 2020 -2025
Make Every Bite Count With the Dietary Guidelines.
https://www.dietaryguidelines.gov/sites/default/files/202
1-03/Dietary_Guidelines_for_Americans-2020-2025.pdf

USDA. (n.d.). Eat fish! Which fish? That fish! Go fish!
https://aglab.ars.usda.gov/fuel-your-
curiosity/aquaculture/eat-fish-which-fish-that-fish-go-
fish/

Varady, K. A. (2011). Intermittent versus daily calorie
restriction: which diet regimen is more effective for
weight loss? Obesity Reviews, 12(7), e593–e601.
https://doi.org/10.1111/j.1467-789x.2011.00873.x

Wang, C.-F., Sun, Y.-L., & Zang, H.-X. (2014). Music therapy
improves sleep quality in acute and chronic sleep
disorders: A meta-analysis of 10 randomized studies.
International Journal of Nursing Studies, 51(1), 51–62.
https://doi.org/10.1016/j.ijnurstu.2013.03.008

Wang, Y., Mei, H., Jiang, Y.-R., Sun, W.-Q., Song, Y.-J., Liu, S.-
J., & Jiang, F. (2015). Relationship between Duration of
Sleep and Hypertension in Adults: A Meta-Analysis.
Journal of Clinical Sleep Medicine, 11(09), 1047–1056.
https://doi.org/10.5664/jcsm.5024

World Health Organization. (2016, September 29). Discrimination and negative attitudes about ageing are bad for your health. Www.who.int. https://www.who.int/news/item/29-09-2016-discrimination-and-negative-attitudes-about-ageing-are-bad-for-your-health

World Health Organization. (2020, December 9). The Top 10 Causes of Death. World Health Organization; World Health Organization. https://www.who.int/news-room/fact-sheets/detail/the-top-10-causes-of-death

Xue, L., Zhang, J., Shen, H., Ai, L., & Wu, R. (2020). A randomized controlled pilot study of the effectiveness of magnolia tea on alleviating depression in postnatal women. Food Science & Nutrition, 8(3), 1554–1561. https://doi.org/10.1002/fsn3.1442

Yang, C. L., Schnepp, J., & Tucker, R. M. (2019). Increased Hunger, Food Cravings, Food Reward, and Portion Size Selection after Sleep Curtailment in Women Without Obesity. Nutrients, 11(3), 663. https://doi.org/10.3390/nu11030663

Ye, L., Hutton Johnson, S., Keane, K., Manasia, M., & Gregas, M. (2015). Napping in College Students and Its Relationship With Nighttime Sleep. Journal of American College Health, 63(2), 88–97. https://doi.org/10.1080/07448481.2014.983926

Yeh, P., Walters, A. S., & Tsuang, J. W. (2011). Restless legs syndrome: a comprehensive overview on its epidemiology, risk factors, and treatment. Sleep and Breathing, 16(4), 987–1007. https://doi.org/10.1007/s11325-011-0606-x

Your menstrual cycle | Office on Women's Health. (n.d.). Www.womenshealth.gov. Retrieved May 17, 2022, from https://www.womenshealth.gov/menstrual-cycle/your-menstrual-cycle#:~:text=Your%20menstrual%20cycle.%20A%20menstrual%20cycle%20begins%20with

Zeb, A. (2015). Phenolic profile and antioxidant potential of wild watercress (Nasturtium officinale L.). SpringerPlus, 4(1). https://doi.org/10.1186/s40064-015-1514-5

Zhang, S., Cao, M., & Fang, F. (2020). The Role of Epigallocatechin-3-Gallate in Autophagy and Endoplasmic Reticulum Stress (ERS)-Induced Apoptosis of Human Diseases. Medical Science Monitor : International Medical Journal of Experimental and Clinical Research, 26, e924558-1e924558-12. https://doi.org/10.12659/MSM.924558

Made in the USA
Coppell, TX
21 September 2022

83441659R00115